Girl's Body
And All That Stuff

The Ultimate Book on Everything a Teen or Preteen Needs to Know about Puberty, Periods, Sex Education, and Private Parts for Growing Up!

CLARA ROFFE

Copyright © 2023 by Clara Roffe

All rights reserved. No part of this book may be reproduced in any form or by any electronic or mechanical means, including information storage and retrieval systems, without written permission from the publisher or author, except in the case of a reviewer, who may quote brief passages embodied in critical articles or a review.

This book is a work of fiction. Any references to historical events, real people, or real locales are used fictitiously. All other characters, and all incidents and dialogue, are drawn from the author's imagination and are not to be construed as real.

Table of Contents

INTRODUCTION

CHAPTER ONE

    WHAT IS PUBERTY?
        Physical Changes during Puberty
        Mental and Emotional Changes during Puberty
        How to Describe Physical and Emotional Changes

CHAPTER TWO

    WHAT ARE PRIVATE PARTS?
        Anatomy of the Female Private Parts
            How to Talk About Private Parts
        How to Care for Private Parts
            Teaching Your Daughter about Personal Hygiene
            Teaching Your Daughter about the Importance of Wearing Clean Underwear
            Teaching Your Daughter about the Dangers of Abusing Her Private Parts

CHAPTER THREE

    SEXTING AND SEX EDUCATION
        How to Have a Sexual Conversation with Your Girl
        Educating Your Girl about the Value of Modesty
    PROTECTING YOUR GIRL FROM SEXUAL PREDATORS

CHAPTER FOUR

    GOOD TOUCH, BAD TOUCH. WHAT THEY ARE ALL ABOUT?

CHAPTER FIVE

    PUBERTY PROBLEMS WHILE GROWING UP
        Acne during Puberty
        Girls' Practical Acne Treatments
        Teen anxiety and the puberty blues: a nightmare for parents
        Autism Spectrum Disorders
        The Connection: Thyroid Problems and Puberty

CHAPTER SIX

    HOW SPORTS CAN HELP TO IMPROVE A GIRL'S SELF-ESTEEM
    THE VALUE OF TAKING A YOUNG GIRL TO A GYNECOLOGIST

CHAPTER SEVEN

DISCUSSING A GIRL'S FIRST PERIOD
  What is the Right Age to Start Talking to Your Girl about Menstruation?
  How to Predict the Arrival of Your Daughter's First Period
  Getting Your Girl Ready for Her Period
  Her First Period

CHAPTER EIGHT

BREAST AND BRA
  Your Daughter's Health & Breast Growth
  What Your Young Girl Should Know About Bra Types
  Examining Young Girls' Risk for Breast Cancer and Self-Protection Strategies

CHAPTER NINE

CHOOSING THE RIGHT FOODS
  10 Surprising Methods for Raising a Healthy Eater: Real Food, Real Kids, and Real Love
  A Teenage Girl's Guide to 50 Safe Pounds of Weight Loss
  Teenage girls' extreme diets

CONCLUSION

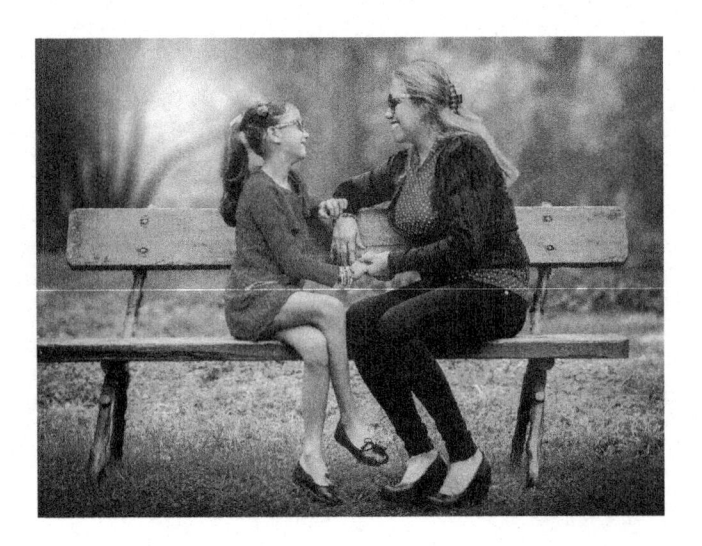

Introduction

Growing up, I didn't understand the significance of the changes I was experiencing. I was a young girl, and suddenly my body was going through so many changes that I didn't understand. I had no idea that I was going through puberty.

My body was growing and changing in ways I couldn't control. I was developing breasts, growing taller, and my skin was getting oilier. I was also getting my period for the first time, which was a massive shock to my system. I had no idea what was going on and why these changes were happening to me.

I began to feel like I was on an unexpected journey, and I had no idea where it would take me or how to get through it. I had many questions, but I was too embarrassed to ask them. I felt like I was the only person going through these changes and that no one else could understand what I was going through.

I tried to talk to my friends and family, but they couldn't relate to my experiences. I felt alone and confused. I was also scared of the changes and the unknown. I was worried about how my body would look and how others would perceive me.

Eventually, I found solace in books, magazines, and articles about puberty and started to understand what was happening to my body and why. I also learned to take care of my changing body by eating healthy, exercising, and using skincare products.

Learning about puberty helped me to feel more confident and empowered. I thought I had some control over the changes happening to me, and I was no longer scared of the unknown. I accepted the changes and embraced them as part of my journey.

Puberty can be an unexpected journey, but it doesn't have to be scary. With the correct information and support, you can make the experience positive. I'm so glad I was able to learn about puberty and understand the changes happening to me, which helped me become the person I am today.

Our inner maiden is left hanging, waiting, and uncertain because most of us mothers are not welcomed into womanhood. As mothers, we promise to give our daughters a different experience, only to witness them fleeing! What is incorrect about this image?

The first step toward empowering and embracing your daughter as a woman is to address YOUR inner maiden, who may not have felt empowered or welcomed when you reached adulthood.

Rarely is the tale of menarche, the beginning of our period told. It's interesting to see how women tend to talk about everything with one another, from their first sexual experiences to their triumphs and tragedies.

As women, we've come a long way. We started acting firmly. By passing "glass ceilings," we combined motherhood with our careers and we choose whether or not to have children. We can accomplish anything, but do we savor the cycle that is the foundation of our womanhood?

You still carry inside of you the adolescent girl who may not have been accepted into womanhood, dormant and waiting. Except for the fact that you may experience menstrual cramps, detest your periods, or consider them "a nuisance," "a bother," or "the curse," you are largely unaware of her presence.

You have a coming-of-age girl waiting inside of you, just like Sleeping Beauty. However, no Sleeping Beauty is coming to wake you up. This work is internal. YOURS!

So how do you start? **As Albert Einstein once said, you must approach a problem with a different mindset than what produced it.** Being heard and seen is the solution because the pain was created. By making you invisible and ignoring your needs as a girl coming of age.

Set aside time to share your period experience with one or more of your close female friends. The feelings of relief, solace, and camaraderie that this straightforward act inspires will astound you. Your health and strength as a fully integrated woman lies in breaking this silence. It also marks the beginning of your daughter's transition into womanhood.

I journeyed from disliking my period to reclaiming it as my spiritual fulcrum. The key to arousing the Sleeping Beauty inside us is sharing our period stories and creating safe spaces for other women to do the same.

Share your first-period story with a close female friend in your living room, cafes, park benches, or any other place where women congregate to support one another through conversation. You can start today by taking this action to reclaim the entirety of your "woman being." Additionally, it is a crucial first step in getting you ready for your daughter's coming of age!

Is your daughter getting close to puberty? Is she there already?

Then it would be best if you read this book from chapter one.

Chapter One

What is Puberty?

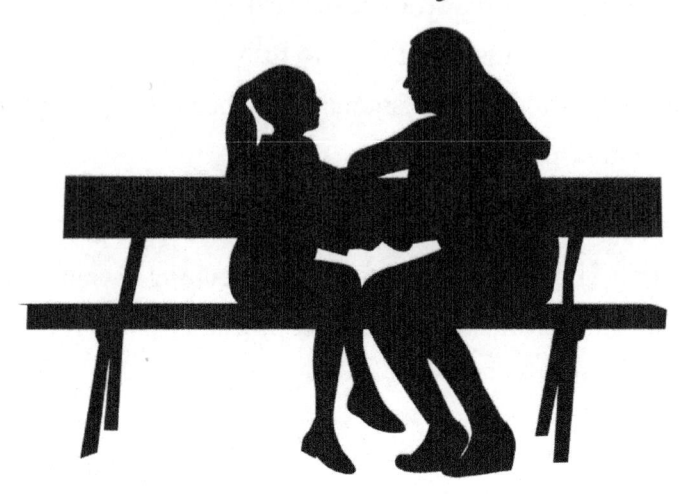

When a child reaches puberty, their body gradually changes to resemble that of a young adult. These modifications go far. Physical development typically happens quickly, and the change from child to tall, gangly youth can occasionally seem to happen almost instantly. In this change, girls are slightly more precocious than boys.

For girls, adolescent physical changes often start around age eleven (or even earlier), whereas for boys, they usually start around age thirteen. Throughout the majority of their time in high school, girls maintain this relative advantage over boys, but by the time they enter college, the distinction has vanished. Girls typically date boys who are just a little older than they are, and this tendency is likely to last into adulthood. Women eventually tend to marry men who are a little older than they are.

Growth in height is the most obvious of a young person's extensive physical changes during adolescence.

However, some young people continue to grow taller well into their early twenties. Full height can be reached as early as the fourteenth year. The timing and rate of development of the endocrine glands, which include the ovaries and testes, are among the factors that determine this (the gonads). Many of the maturational changes associated with puberty are brought on by the hormones secreted by these glands, which also prevent height growth. Growth stops early if puberty is quick and the physical changes are finished early. Height growth might take longer if the gonads take longer to mature.

Girls go through puberty and start to take on the shape of young women. They lose their earlier resemblance to the more boyish figure of childhood as the breasts grow, the hips enlarge, and so on. The uterus, one of a woman's vital internal organs, develops during this time, and the first period is a clear indication that she is about to reach sexual maturity. This can happen as early as age ten, but it can also wait until age thirteen or even fourteen. Girls need to be ready for this occasion. The mother, who should speak directly to her daughter about body composition and function, is the best person to start this preparation. Otherwise, she might hear or fantasize about false and distorted information from other girls.

The emergence of secondary sexual traits signals the beginning of adolescence.

The growth of pubic and axillary hair are two obvious examples. When a boy develops a beard, it is necessary to make an initial effort to shave; however, regular grooming becomes necessary as the facial hair grows heavier. The boy's genitalia is getting close to adult size, and emissions show testicular development and fertility. Another obvious secondary characteristic is the deepening of the voice, which is most noticeable in boys.

Adolescent skin goes through distinctive changes the development of mature sweat glands and an increase in skin oiliness Acne appears frequently, especially in people with fair skin, and when severe, it greatly distresses the adolescent. The adolescent is particularly sensitive to anything that might be seen as a flaw or imperfection. Adolescent acne can occasionally result in severe emotional distress. Even though the condition is only temporary, if careful skin care alone is unable to control it, psychiatric guidance and assistance may be required.

The adolescent boy's development of sexual fertility and the accompanying sexual urges almost always result in the practice of masturbation. Adolescents' first sexual experiences are typically masturbatory.

Parents should never try to alarm adolescents with unfounded stories of harmful consequences (which are nonexistent) or with feelings of guilt or remorse. Adolescents are unlikely to need explanations or interference from adults regarding masturbation. The adolescent boy is biologically and sexually capable of becoming a father, but he is not emotionally prepared to do so, even if society were to approve of it, which it rarely does before the boy is at least 18 years old. Thus, the boy's only available sexual outlet in which he can indulge without involving or upsetting others is masturbation.

When a girl experiences physical changes like menstruation, she typically feels happy and proud of herself. She starts to feel that she is getting closer to the dignity of womanhood, just like the older girls she looks up to and, if they have a good relationship, just like her mother. This self-confidence, however, can only be attained if she can foresee that her impending womanliness will bring about a positive promise for the future through proper teaching and modeling in her own home. The changes in adolescence cause anxiety and confusion in many adolescent girls. If a girl is not given the support she needs to understand and accept her approach to adult femininity, she may foolishly try to hide or deny her physical development. Masturbation can occasionally develop into a habit. Daughters' adolescent doubts about these roles frequently reflect the disturbed attitudes of women toward the roles of wife and mother. The wholesome mother imparts to her daughter her assurance that the social, familial, and sexual responsibilities of being a wife and mother are profoundly satisfying.

Boys experience great fulfillment and pride when they grow to be big and strong, capable of feats of physical prowess that they both admire in others and themselves. A boy with early football player physical development is likely to have it easier in some ways than a boy with minimal physical development. Boys typically compare themselves to others harshly and are especially sensitive to anything that might imply they are less capable than their friends, especially in sports. Boys tend to be particular about the size of their chest expansion, the power of their arms, and their general appearance. Some of them go to great lengths to correct what they view as physical flaws. For many insecure teenagers, having wide hips, skinny or fat legs, or round or flat breasts are issues that cause them unwarranted anxiety.

Boys and girls occasionally need to have their competitive feelings expressed in worries about their abilities and appearance directly addressed. When given the chance, the adolescent will inquire about physical changes and express his uncertainty and worry about how well he will compare to people his age. An approach to the seemingly straightforward issue of how he feels about his own body and appearance will frequently lead to a frank discussion of deeper-lying concerns about his sexual impulses and his social and vocational uncertainties because most adolescent anxieties center on the problem of his ability to meet the demands of adult life.

Physical Changes during Puberty

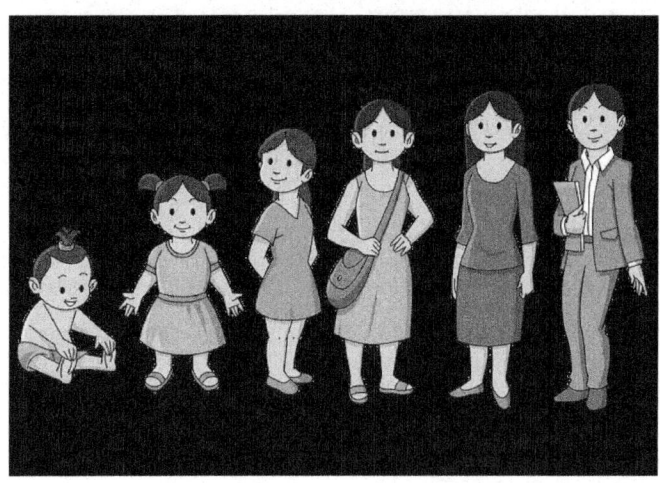

In time, little girls will develop into young ladies. During these formative years, a girl will experience various changes during puberty, particularly in terms of her physical appearance. Their bodies will undergo a variety of changes that will show they are developing into young ladies. These changes don't need to worry you, girls; they are just the way things are. All girls will go through these physical transformations. One of a young girl's most eagerly anticipated experiences is puberty.

For girls, puberty lasts for several years. Girls will experience completely uncontrollable physical and even emotional changes during this time. This is so that the changes can be attributed to the hormones and chemicals that the body produces as a result. A girl's breast size increases during puberty, which is the most obvious physical change. The girl typically experiences this when she is between the ages of 8 and 13. The girl will then be required to wear a brassiere during this time.

In addition, hair will begin to grow on various body parts. As the waist gets smaller and the hips get wider, the body will begin to take shape. Additionally, the stomach and legs will begin to enlarge. Simply put, this indicates that the young girl is becoming a woman. Along with these physical modifications, the girl will also start to see more acne developing on their face, back, and chest. Whiteheads, blackheads, and pimples are all common teenage skin issues. One only needs to consult a dermatologist if these skin issues have gotten out of control.

A girl must wear various pairs of pants during these times. They will have to stop wearing the baby pants they are currently wearing as a result. Since their hips will soon expand, they should purchase a size larger than usual. Menstruation will begin at this time as well. They need to be aware of the proper way to handle this condition. Some people who have the condition might experience pain. Even dysmenorrhea would be present. On what to do during one's period, one should be advised.

A girl will learn how to use sanitary napkins and perhaps how to remove period stains once she reaches puberty. Just a few of the topics a girl will learn about during puberty are those mentioned above. Daughters should be guided by their parents, especially their mothers so that puberty comes and goes smoothly for them. Girls go through a stage where they experience a range of feelings that they are unable to control. With the support and guidance of their parents, girls won't ever have to fear going through puberty.

Mental and Emotional Changes during Puberty

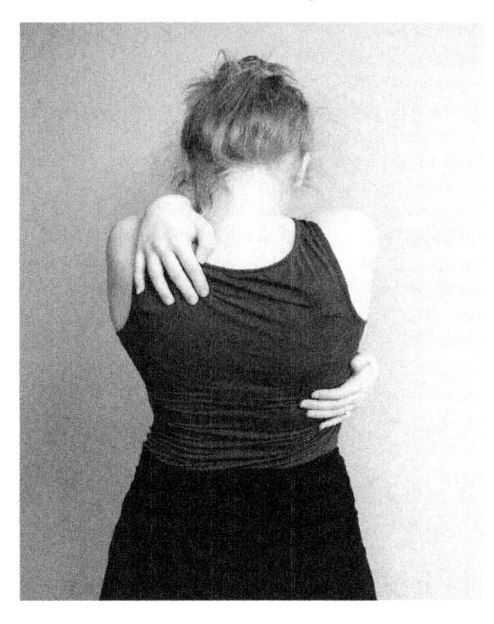

Raging hormones may interfere with adolescent emotions as the body develops. Although there are many physical changes associated with puberty, it's also common for young girls to go through emotional changes as well. Most emotional changes that occur during puberty are reflected in the way that they behave. It can be challenging for parents as well as teenagers to adjust to these changes in their appearance and emotional state. A child transitions from a child to a sexually mature adult during puberty. Adolescence is best described as an emotional roller coaster ride.

Puberty starts with an increase in hormone production, which generates changes that influence both the body and the psyche. The growth, development, and operation of the sexual organs, bones, brain, and skin are all directly impacted by hormonal changes. They also increase libido, one of the main emotional catalysts during adolescence.

Boys and girls both go through puberty around the age of 11 or 12, with girls going through it around the age of 10 or 11.

Puberty can, however, start early or late for both boys and girls. Their social and domestic interactions are impacted by this. Males and females experience different biological or physical changes, but emotional and cognitive changes are generally similar. Teenage boys and girls both experience mood swings as a result of these changes. Children have a wide spectrum of emotions, and because their bodies and emotions are actively influenced by active hormones, they have many questions and uncertainties about who they are and what they are experiencing. They need all the support and direction their parents and guardians can give them at this time because they are most vulnerable. Although it won't be simple, your adolescent must listen and be there for them when they need you to ease the transition and reduce stress for everyone.

Understanding what your adolescent child experiences during that time and how you can support her will help you make adolescence more enjoyable and less stressful for her. The list of emotional changes your child will probably go through during puberty is provided below.

- Physically altered modifications.

Secondary sexual organs begin to develop in the body as puberty sets in. The development of breasts, curves, and facial hair in girls, as well as the appearance of facial hair (a larger Adam's apple), are examples of outwardly visible changes that can occur.

- Girls start gaining weight, expanding their shoulders, and building stronger muscles.
- Girls also begin their period and develop pubic hair.
- One of the most important biological changes that take place during puberty is brain development.
- Their primary sexual organs' levels of secretion have an impact on how much of these changes occur. This would imply that some children might be tall for their age, some might grow little facial hair, and others might have more facial hair than they desire.
- Teenagers going through puberty will also be concerned about acne, also known as pimples.
- Children who develop their sexuality too early may even encounter bullying or taunting at school.

A child may find changes in the body frightening and confusing, especially if they don't understand what is happening. Your kids may become self-conscious and believe they have a problem if you don't make them aware of it. It becomes worse when they avoid discussing it and begin to worry.

How to Manage This:

To help kids deal with the physical changes they are going through effectively, it's important to be aware of them. As their children approach puberty, parents must discuss these changes with them. Giving them books that are suitable for their age can be a nice addition to talking with them because it gives them a chance to investigate and discover the changes on their own.

Encourage them to discuss their fears and ask any questions they may have. Your daughter may find it difficult and even awkward to discuss her sexual changes and feelings, but it is your responsibility as a parent to help her feel comfortable doing so. Subtly and in a way that captures their interest, introduce the subject. Do not pressure them to discuss it because doing so will only increase their anxiety. Discuss it at their speed rather than yours.

Give your teen a healthy diet and encourage them to participate in sports and physical activity and they will get healthier and feel so much better about themselves.

- Mood swings, emotional outbursts, crying fits, and aggression.

Adolescents frequently experience mood swings. The hormonal changes in their bodies are typically responsible for the subtle changes in their feelings and emotions. Your girl will exhibit varying degrees of composure and reasoned behavior.

Puberty-affected teenagers are at risk. They might be easily agitated, overly emotional, and easily excited. They may spend hours sobbing over seemingly unimportant issues and become overly enthusiastic about things that adults might find annoying.

Teenagers experience a range of strong emotions, including anger so much so that you might occasionally think they despise you. It can be confusing and overwhelming to experience so many different emotions at once.

This causes annoyance and rage, which manifest as aggression and, in rare instances, violence. Regarding the significant developmental changes that go along with an emerging sense of self and self-identity, it can be helpful to imagine that your girl shares a lot in common with a toddler. The teen, however, might be larger than you. It is no longer possible to physically restrain them to help them control their strong emotions. They do, however, need the restraint that your composed emotional presence and explicit limit-setting provide.

How to Manage This:

It takes emotional maturity to live a healthy life. Emotional IQ is a skill that we acquire over time. It is your duty as a parent to assist your child in navigating the ups and downs of their emotions.

Never forget that changes in hormone levels are largely to blame for these emotional changes. As a result, your child's extreme mood swings are typically brought on by that. If you can support your child during this frequently difficult time, it will pass as they enter the young adult stage. The best way to handle these mood swings is to calmly listen and refrain from responding in kind. Don't respond angrily if your child snaps at you. Consider for a moment what might be causing them to act in that manner. Additionally, it gives your kid a chance to settle down.

Clear the air by discussing what they did or said without using an accusatory tone. Let them know that if they ever feel overwhelmed or confused, they can always talk to you.

Set a good example for your teen by responding healthily and maturely to her. Always strive to maintain composure and common sense in their presence.

- Identity Crisis: Self-Awareness.

One is neither a child nor an adult during adolescence and puberty, children begin to feel and behave differently. They become aware of the changes taking place in their bodies. Girls, who typically mature more quickly than boys, are particularly affected by this.

Teenagers may tend to compare their bodies to those of others and link their sense of self-worth with it and they make an effort to identify their preferences. It's time to explore new interests and deepen your understanding of who you are to discover your unique qualities.

The pressure to fit in also contributes to people's efforts to discover who they are. They might ponder whether they should associate with the most popular people or those with whom they feel most at ease. They debate whether they ought to join the math club or the soccer team.

How to Manage This:

Teenagers may look up to their parents at this stage, but they also develop role models outside the family, like a friend or a famous person, and strive to be like them in some way. In other words, your daughter needs a mentor to help her develop as a person. If you and your girl get along well, she might aspire to be just like you or your spouse. It's typical for independent or even rebellious kids to look outside the home for role models.

You should keep a close eye on them and be aware of the decisions they make and the significant relationships they have outside the home. When necessary, you should also offer advice.

- Modification of Relationships.

The dynamics of relationships change quickly after puberty. Your child might begin to spend more time with their friends than with you. They might even feel ashamed to be seen in public with a parent. Your child might value their friends more than their family. This behavior is typical and a necessary component of a healthy separation process.

Both friends and family are significant to adolescents. Along with parental guidance and support, they desire the approval of their peers. Therefore, forcing them into a decision where they must pick one over the other will not be helpful. It will increase their anxiety and might even paint the parent as a bad guy who wants to dominate them. They might eventually begin to doubt and reject what their parents say and do.

How to Manage This:

It's possible that adolescents won't always follow adult instructions. At times, they might come off as disrespectful and rebellious. Whether or not they are mature enough, adolescents are independent and want to make their own decisions. Rather than outright rejecting their independence, try to establish a manageable collaborative relationship.

Instead of telling them that they are no longer children, teach them about responsibility and what is expected of them. Allow them to hang out with their friends as well, but keep an eye on their activities to keep them from running afoul of the law. Again, the idea of providing options that you used when your children were toddlers is applicable in this situation.

Establish clear ground rules for your family's conduct, interaction, and socialization. By doing this, you can teach your kids about boundaries and stop them from experimenting with risky activities.

- Sensitive to everything.

Children become extremely sensitive to certain things during puberty due to hormonal changes. Being rejected by a boy can feel like the end of the world, and even a small zit or spot of acne on their face can seem like a major catastrophe. What's worse is that you no longer understand what triggers your adolescent's anger. Additionally, this is the time when the adolescent is most open to outside influences.

How to Manage This:

Keeping your cool when interacting with an overly emotional teen is challenging. It is more difficult to counsel emotionally sensitive teenagers because they are prone to feeling overwhelmed and are unable to understand logical reasoning.

Don't lecture your child if they are feeling weak. Instead, give them space to express their emotions while you listen to them. Tell them you understand what they're going through and that you're available to help if she needs it, to show them that you care.

- Your kid might experience confusion.

During puberty, your girl goes through a lot of novel feelings and sensations. They might feel uneasy and even disturbed by the physical changes that occur and the novel emotions that result from them. If you don't address it, your girl might believe that something is wrong with you.

How to Manage This:

Children who feel like there is a problem with them feel under pressure to fix it, which can result in emotional problems like distorted body images. When your child understands that the feelings are normal and have nothing to be ashamed of, she might not feel as awkward. You can even describe how you felt when you were going through that phase to help them a little.

- Lack of confidence and indecision.

Teenagers are between adults and children. Teenagers frequently feel uncertain about their place in the world and the position they should adopt as a result and they feel emotions like fear, insecurity, and helplessness just like children do, but they also feel like they shouldn't because they are adults. Indecision is frequently a result of this uncertainty.

As they get older, kids are also expected to act or behave in a certain way. They must exercise responsibility as well. Additionally, the shift in expectations can be extremely perplexing.

How to Manage This:

Change is a good thing, but it shouldn't be forced upon someone. Recognize that puberty is a gradual process and that when it occurs, you are interacting with a person who is both a child and an adult. Don't expect your child to change on its own once puberty begins.

Help them gradually adjust to the demands and changes that come with them. Give them small, responsible tasks, but don't count on them to complete them correctly the first time. Give them time to gradually adjust to that role.

- Sexual inclinations and gendered behaviors.

Children experience sexual feelings because of the spike in sex hormones that occurs during puberty. Your child develops new emotions and perspectives as they approach sexual maturity.

Additionally, they might begin exhibiting gender-specific mannerisms. For instance, your little girl might begin expressing interest in clothing, cosmetics, and other feminine items. These, however, differ significantly based on personality traits but your child may be investigating their gender identity and sexual orientation.

Your daughter might start considering dating, and their perspective on their peers who are of the other sex may also change. When they watch a romantic scene on television, they might become aroused and attracted to the other sex. At this point in her development, your girl might realize she has feelings for her same-sex partner.

How to Manage This:

While a child's sexual development begins to mature during puberty, this does not necessarily indicate that your children are considering having sex. They only have feelings of a sexual nature, which is confusing.

It's time to talk to your child about sex and sexuality if they're discussing dates or asking you about them. The most crucial aspect is to avoid making them feel uncomfortable or guilty about how they are feeling.

- Peer pressure increases the desire to fit in.

Teenagers are delicate, susceptible to peer pressure, and constantly feel the need to fit in. Teenagers feel pressured to go above and beyond to win their peers' approval, which motivates them to alter their social behavior, speech patterns, and modes of dress. To fit in, they might occasionally choose the wrong path.

As a result of spending more time with friends than you, your child's behavior will change. To be "cool," they might feel pressured to experiment with new behaviors like smoking, drinking, or even using drugs.

How to Manage This:

Peer pressure cannot be removed. You can, however, reassure your child that they are not required to follow their desires to fit in or be deemed "cool." Encourage them to grow into their distinct personalities and to speak up for their convictions. Help them understand what they stand to gain or lose if they follow peer pressure, and then give them the freedom to choose and help them, but don't make decisions for them.

- Differing Opinions

A conflict of interest may occasionally arise due to your adolescent's confusion and indecision during the transitional period. For instance, an adult may want to exercise independence and go to the movies with friends, whereas the child within them may want to go to a movie with the parents.

How to Manage This:

Conflicting ideas can be problematic because they put the adolescent in a challenging situation. They may feel compelled to make a decision and under pressure to do so without causing harm to anyone.

When your child must decide between an outing with their parents and one with their friends, assure them that there is no wrong decision. They can choose to do whatever brings them the most joy. Most of the time, allowing them the freedom of choice also helps them develop their sense of justice and judgment, which helps them choose the best course of action.

- Your girl may prefer to be by herself.

Teenagers go through a transitional time during puberty and attempt to make their judgments. Despite your best efforts to engage them in conversation and collaboration, they frequently request your respect for their privacy. This behavior is expected, but if your child spends a lot of time alone, it may be a sign that they are having more difficulties than is usual for their developmental stage.

How to Manage This:

Teenagers' desire to isolate themselves is common. However, it is cause for concern if you believe they are spending too much time alone in the room rather than with friends or family. Discuss it with your teen and understand why they prefer to be alone. Additionally, learn what they do on their own, and be subtle in your approach. You might want to consult a professional if you believe it to be a problem area.

Teenagers' emotional shifts are not abnormal. However, if you observe that they are acting strangely, engaging in hazardous behavior, experiencing academic issues, or having difficulty in their relationships both within and outside of the house, you may decide to seek out professional support and guidance.

How to Describe Physical and Emotional Changes

Your autistic child will eventually go through puberty. Even though it can be challenging for a child without a disability and their parents, it can be especially challenging for a child with a disability like autism.

How do you explain to a child with autism who struggles with communication and comprehension how and why their bodies and feelings are changing so drastically during puberty? Due to their significant physical changes, which can be extremely traumatic for girls if they don't understand them, they may face an even greater challenge.

Get rid of fears and myths.

This can be a very difficult situation for some cultures and religious beliefs because it may be considered taboo to discuss such subjects.

It's time to discard these beliefs, though, if you want to survive this with your child. As a parent or caregiver of a child with an autism spectrum disorder, you must adopt the stance that you must educate the child about the changes well in advance and make an effort to help them comprehend, or at the very least be ready for, what is about to happen.

If you think about it logically, it is only natural; it is a part of who we are. Although it is regarded as a very private matter, you must make every effort to help the child feel comfortable talking about it. This holds for kids without disabilities.

Information and Guidance

Although they vary from state to state and country to country, some disability services can assist and/or guide with advice and reading material on the best ways to help the child understand puberty but always try to learn as much as you can. Don't be afraid; it's just a normal part of life. Try to always see it that way.

Our daughter experienced the "puberty blues," but thanks to the fact that I'm her mom and I have the foresight and a no-nonsense approach, it was not a problem. We can speak from experience and pass on information that helped us.

Get autistic children ready.

In the end, my daughter experienced no surprises; everything went exactly as she had read about, been told about, and been braced for.

The preparation was well worth it because she can now take care of herself in that regard.

For boys, it's essentially the same; it might not be as difficult because their circumstances call for less effort, but the same principles still hold. Preparation and comprehension will help people deal with changes when they happen because they will be prepared for them.

Planning and preparation are the key elements to everything when dealing with children on the autism spectrum, as we frequently advise. You must give them plenty of time to process the information and feel confident about the decision.

Chapter Two

What are Private Parts?

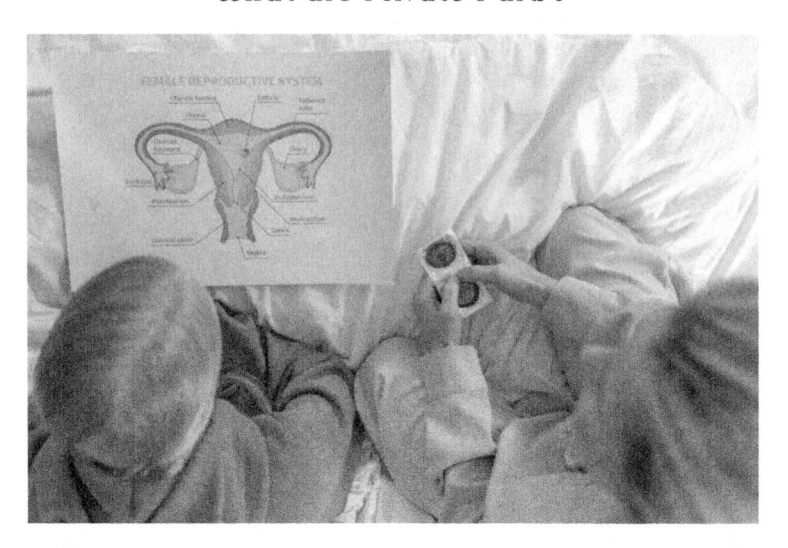

Human Private Parts are body parts that are typically not visible to the public and are generally considered to be sensitive or intimate including primary sexual organs or other parts of the body that are not typically exposed to the public. Private parts are considered private and seen as a source of personal privacy and modesty.

The meaning of private parts has changed over time. In many cultures, private parts are seen as something to be kept hidden, and exposure of them is seen as shameful or forbidden. In some cultures, exposure to private parts is seen as a sign of disrespect or even as a form of sexual misconduct. In the West, there is an increasing acceptance of the exposure of private parts in the media, and this often comes with a certain level of objectification of the body.

This topic is also culturally and historically dependent. In some cultures, private parts are seen as something to be respected and kept sacred, while in others they are seen as something to be exposed to and celebrated. In Western cultures, private parts are often seen as hidden, while in Eastern cultures they are often seen as something to be displayed.

Depending on some contexts, such as in medical examinations or sexual activity, private parts may be seen as something to be explored and appreciated, while in other contexts, such as in public settings, private parts may be seen as something to be kept hidden.

At the same time, private parts can also serve as a source of pleasure, identity, and even power. Private parts can be seen as a way to assert one's autonomy and independence and can be seen as a source of empowerment or even as a form of self-expression.

This is therefore highly personal and context-dependent. Whether private parts are seen as something to be kept hidden or exposed depends on the culture, context, and individual. What is considered private will vary from person to person, and in some cases, private parts can be seen as a source of pleasure, identity, or even power?

Anatomy of the Female Private Parts

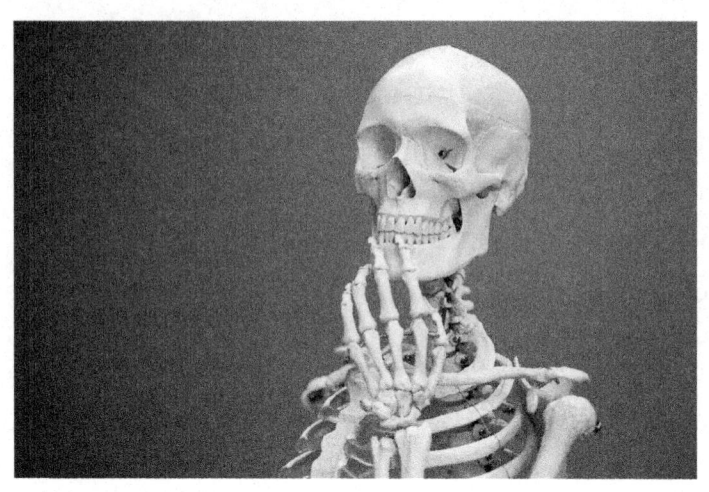

1. Vulva

The vulva starts over her pubic bone and extends far back between her legs, not far from the opening of her cervix. The vulva starts relatively high up, at the lowest part of the belly, in young girls or some women. The vulva is frequently pushed lower between the legs as the pubic bone grows during development.

The outer genital lips, also known as the great lips or the Labia majora, are the most noticeable features of the vulva.

The clitoris, a structure resembling a knob with a hood reminiscent of the penile foreskin, is located between the upper portions of the lips. The Labia minora, or small or inner genital lips, are located beneath the clitoris and extend to the clitoral foreskin. These encircle the vaginal vestibule, a receded region. The vaginal opening is located directly below the urethral opening in the vaginal vestibule.

- **The Area between the Lips and the Genital Lips**

The labia majora extend backward between the woman's legs, where they also join, and meet at the lower portion of the belly, just over the pubic bone. The labia minora, or inner lips, vary greatly in size and shape. They may lie entirely within the region of the great lips or project outward from it.

Sebaceous glands on the inside of the genital lips secrete an oily liquid, and there are also sweat glands that produce salty secretions. Sebum is created when this fluid combines with fatty skin cells that are shed from the inner surface of the lips and helpful bacteria. Sebum serves as both a lubricant and a protector.

- **The Glands of the Urethra and Para urethra**

The urinary opening is located in the vestibule, some distance from the clitoris; on occasion, it is even positioned at the upper rim of the vaginal opening. It is situated between the inner lips. On either side of the urethra, there are two glands known as Skene's glands or Paraurethral glands that secrete fluid similar to that of the male prostate. The glands tend to empty themselves before and during orgasm, which can help explain why some women experience female ejaculation.

The urethral orifice is immediately beneath the vaginal opening. In Jung girls, the majority of its closure is provided by a thin membrane known as the hymen. At some point, the hymen will rupture, leaving only remnants at the edge of the vaginal opening. The uterus, or womb, is reached through the vagina.

The inner vaginal wall is made up of a sheet of elastic connective tissue covered by epithelium, and a sheet of muscles surrounds that. Numerous glands secrete a lubricating slime in the vaginal wall tissue. Just before and during puberty, this secretion tends to increase. It occurs all the time but increases during sexual excitement.

Although few nerves in the vaginal wall can recognize sensations, it does have nerve endings that regulate glands and muscles.

The Bartholin's glands, which are located on both sides of the vagina and fairly far back, secrete a slime, especially right before the female orgasm. Additionally, this secretion might help women ejaculate.

- **The Erectile and Clitoris Bodies**

Like the penis, the clitoris has a hood that can be continuous with the minor lips or extend downward on both sides of the minor lips to give the impression that the woman has even more lips. Like the penis, the visible clitoris can become blood-filled, engorged, and erect.

It has a set of erectile bodies that extend inside the vulva's structural elements in addition to the clitoris, giving the vulva as a whole the capacity to become engorged with blood. The erectile bodies are made up of an elastic connective tissue framework and a mesh of blood vessels.

In the lower portion of the clitoris, you'll find the erectile body corpus bulbospongiosus.

The urethra and vagina are framed by this body, which splits into two branches, the vestibule bulbs. These two great bodies continue on either side of the vaginal vestibule the bulbospongiosus muscle, which surrounds these bodies in part.

The erectile bodies, or corpora cavernosa, which each extend inside as two bodies and are known as the clitoris' legs, are located in the upper part of the clitoris. These are located beneath each of the great lips along the inner rim of the pubic bone. The ischiocavernosus muscle partially encircles these bodies as well.

The entire clitoris is covered in a very dense density of nerve endings. Numerous of these are housed in tiny bodies of connective tissue that can transmit and concentrate impulses like pressure and vibration toward the nerve endings.

- **The Vulva's G-Spot and Internal Sensory Areas**

The upper vaginal wall is reached by a sensitive structure that descends on both sides of the urethra from the clitoris and has a swampy appearance due to a network of blood vessels. Pressure, vibration, or stimulation from within the vagina can stimulate this structure from the clitoral side. The "G-spot" is the area of this structure that is closest to the vaginal wall.

Sensations in the clitoris and throughout the entire structure, all the way to the vaginal wall, play a part in a woman's orgasm. When the clitoris is where the majority of the sensations are felt, the orgasm is known as a clitoral orgasm. Sometimes, the majority of sensations are felt over the vaginal wall, which is referred to as the "G-spot" or the "vaginal orgasm."

- **The Vulva's Nervation and Blood Supply**

The perineal nerve, a branch of the pudendal nerve, is a nerve that regulates numerous significant functions in the pelvic area and innervates the clitoris and the central portions of the vulva. The posterior femoral cutaneous nerves, which also control the surfaces of the thighs, have branches that control the peripheral vulva. These nerves have parasympathetic fibers that regulate glands, blood vessels, and involuntary muscle movements in addition to fibers that transmit sensations and control the vulva's voluntary muscles.

Internal pudendal arteries on both sides of the vulva supply a significant portion of the vulva's blood supply. This artery has branches that travel to the rectum, labia, clitoral region, and other parts of the pelvic region.

2. Vagina

The delicate, brittle tissue that makes up the vagina is easily torn when dry. The same kind of skin and tissue that make up the vagina also make up the human lips. Lips are delicate, brittle, and prone to tearing. When kissed, they swell and engorge. When they are bruised, they turn red. Similar types of tissue make up the vagina.

It's amazing how elastic the vagina is. Babies go through it, even though I know you'd rather not think about it. A head can pass through the cervix when it opens up sufficiently. The truth is that the vagina is an amazing body part certainly not what you want to think of when you think of one.

There are many ways that vaginas distinguish men from boys (I mean women). Men cannot give birth; only women can do so. We have some unique body parts. I've gathered a ton of knowledge about the vagina. While some of these may not come as a surprise to you, the majority will.

- There are over 8,000 nerve endings in the vagina but I apologize, there are only 4,000 in boys. Given how frequently you discuss your privates, I wanted to make sure you were aware of how delicate the vagina is.
- The typical vagina measures 3 to 4 inches long. When sexually aroused, it can expand by 200 percent.
- Like a man's penis, the vagina is made of erectile tissue. When aroused, it becomes engorged and swells like the penis.
- It is a closed system, the vagina. The cervix, which opens during childbirth, is located at the top end. The stomach does not receive anything from the vagina.
- Squalene is secreted by the vagina like a shark. Unsettling, huh?

Girl's Body And All That Stuff | 41

- The vagina and labia are not protected from STDs by a condom. Herpes and warts can develop if the labia touch the scrotum.
- The lips, or labia minora, are typically 3/4" long. Of the 2981 women who were measured, yes. Some are uneven, some are inside, and some hang. Each of them is ideal just the way they are.
- The delicate vagina was intended to be protected by pubic hair. To entice a mate, it captures the scent of the vagina. There's a reason why you shouldn't shave it, girls!
- In 30% of women, only sexual contact can cause orgasms and to orgasm, most women require clitoral stimulation.
- There are numerous nerve endings in the clitoris. The clitoris has twice as many nerve endings as the penis and it can be as small as a pea or as long as seven inches. Similar to the penis, it enlarges when aroused.
- A woman will squirt fluid and ejaculate during a G-Spot orgasm. This isn't feces. The fluid, which is created by the Skene glands, resembles the seminal fluid of a man but does not contain sperm. Guys, you don't urinate when you cough, and neither do we. If your woman experiences one of these incredible orgasms, don't shame her. She might be doing it for the last time.
- A woman can experience 11 different kinds of orgasms. Some orgasmic sensations that may occur include clitoral, vaginal, G-Spot, squirting orgasm, A-Spot upper vaginal

wall (anterior fornix), Deep Spot near the cervix (feels like anal sex), breast orgasm, skin orgasm, mental orgasm, and full body orgasm. Yes, we are unique. Maybe I didn't get one.

- The flavor of a woman's vaginal secretion is influenced by whatever she consumes. Vaginal secretions contain a lot of garlic, soy, and onions.
- Contrary to popular belief, the vagina functions like an oven that cleans itself. There is no need for douching.
- Yeast infections brought on by excessive sugar consumption can be treated with probiotics and acidophilus.

3. Uterus

The womb is another name for the uterus. The uterus is where the fetus develops most. As a result, the uterus is an essential component of the female reproductive system. The uterus is hollow and shaped like a pear and a typical uterus has a diameter of several centimeters.

- **Terminal Formation**

The majority of the uterus is made up of myometrium, which is muscles.

The "junctional zone" refers to the myometrium's deepest interior region. Adenomyosis is the term used to describe the process by which this zone thickens during pregnancy. The lining of the uterus is called the endometrium and during menstruation, this lining peels off. The surrounding tissue, known as the parametrium, is typically loose.

☐ Terminal Location

Within the pelvic region, the uterus is situated halfway between the rectum and the bladder. The uterus is where the child develops.

☐ Apartment Sections

The cervix, corpus, fundus, fallopian tubes, ovaries, tissues, endometrium, and myometrium are the eight different parts of a uterus. The first three essentially refer to different uterine regions. The lower part of the uterus is known as the cervix and the middle section of the uterus is called the corpus. Its size and area are both broad. The top part of the uterus is called the fundus and it keeps its dome-like shape. The uterus is divided into five additional sections. To the ovaries are the fallopian tubes. They extend from the uterus' two top sides. The tissues make up the uterus's internal lining. The inner and outer uterine tissue linings are known as the endometrium and myometrium, respectively.

☐ Terminal Function

The uterus serves as the fertilized egg's natural grooming bed. The endometrium receives the implanted egg, also known as an ovum. The blood vessels that are connected to this lining surround the ovum, providing it with nutrition. The ovum develops into a fetus in the uterus, where it then develops into a baby. The enlarged uterus that is carrying the ovum is pushed into the abdomen during pregnancy. The natural driving force behind this process comes from the pelvic region. The uterus mass weighs about a kilogram at these times.

▢ Pregnancy, Uterine Linings, Menstruation, and Tissue

Every month, a typical woman goes through her "fertility" stages. Once a girl reaches puberty, she has reached this significant stage of womanhood. Menstruation is one of the first clear signs of puberty. A mature egg is released by the ovaries during this menstrual stage. The uterus is used to carry the egg. Pregnancy occurs if the egg is fertilized by a male sperm at this time. The uterine tissue linings thicken at this time to protect the fertilized egg and provide a healthy environment for grooming. Menstruation, however, happens if the egg and sperm do not successfully combine. The aforementioned uterine tissue linings begin to separate at this point. The blood that flows out of these uterine linings through the vagina is referred to as the menstruation process.

4. Fallopian Tubes

On either side of the uterus are the fallopian tubes and they keep moving forward, moving toward the ovaries. A fimbria, or finger-like structure, is present at the end of each fallopian tube and extends toward the ovary to catch eggs as they are released. When it's time for ovulation, the fimbria stimulates the ovary. The egg is guided by the fimbria's cilia down the fallopian tube and into the uterus.

The infundibulum is the portion of the fallopian tube that houses the fimbria. The ampulla, a dilated portion of the fallopian tube, is where the infundibulum opens. The ampulla is typically where the fertilization of the egg occurs. After fertilization, the fertilized egg will proceed down the tube's isthmus, which is a smaller section. The intramural oviduct, which is essentially the uterus' entrance, is where it then enters.

Three main layers make fallopian tubes. The mucosa is the first and deepest layer of it. This layer of mucus secretes and shields the tubes. The mucosa has a distinctive appearance that makes it easier to distinguish between the various fallopian tube regions mentioned above. The muscularis externa term for the second layer of the fallopian tubes. Essentially, this layer is made up of muscle tissue that can contract. Through the tubes, the fluid and eggs are moved by these contractions. The serosa is the third layer. This outer lining is slick.

Fallopian tube issues can result in infertility. Infertility is frequently brought on by obstructions, inflammation, and dysfunction of the tubes. Ovaries, fallopian tubes, and/or the uterus are all impacted by pelvic inflammatory disease. An egg's ability to pass through the tube may be blocked by inflammation, which may also reduce the likelihood of a successful pregnancy. Tissues may eventually become glued together as a result of this inflammation, forming a scar. The most frequent reasons for tube blockage are scar tissue and adhesions. Although there are other potential causes, bacterial infections or sexually transmitted diseases are the most frequent causes of pelvic inflammatory disease.

An x-ray can be used to check for tubal occlusion or blockage. The cervix receives an injection of dye. It passes into the fallopian tubes after ascending through the uterus. There isn't a complete blockage in the tube if the dye leaks into the abdominal cavity. The medical term for this process is hysterosalpingogram. The tube itself might not be strong enough to carry an egg to the uterus or there might still be a partial blockage.

A laparoscopy can be done to examine the tubal damage if the fallopian tube is not completely blocked. Your doctor or an infertility specialist may suggest in vitro fertilization or surgery to repair tubal damage occasionally.

5. Ovaries

The female reproductive organs, the ovaries, are located on either side of the uterus. They produce the female reproductive hormones estrogen and progesterone and are responsible for the production of eggs. The ovaries are almond-shaped structures composed of two parts the cortex, which produces the female hormones, and the medulla, which holds the eggs.

These hormones are essential for the development of female secondary sex characteristics, such as breast development and pubic hair. They also regulate the menstrual cycle, preparing the uterus for pregnancy. In addition to hormone production, the ovaries also contain a large number of follicles, which are small sacs filled with immature eggs.

The ovaries are connected to the uterus by the fallopian tubes and when a woman ovulates, a mature egg is released from the ovary and travels through the fallopian tube to the uterus. If the egg is fertilized by a sperm, it will implant in the uterus and a pregnancy will result. If the egg is not fertilized, it will be shed during the woman's next menstrual period.

They are also the source of several other important hormones, including testosterone, luteinizing hormone, and follicle-stimulating hormone. These hormones are important for regulating the menstrual cycle and for reproductive processes such as ovulation.

The ovaries can become diseased or damaged due to a variety of factors, including infection, trauma, or cancer. Diseases of the ovaries can cause infertility, irregular menstrual cycles, or even ovarian cysts. Certain medical conditions, such as polycystic ovary syndrome, can also affect the functioning of the ovaries. In some cases, the ovaries may need to be surgically removed to treat the condition.

Treatment for diseases of the ovaries depends on the cause, but in some cases, surgery may be necessary. It is important to talk to your doctor if your girl has any concerns about her ovaries or reproductive health.

6. Cervix

I am the entrance and the exit. I create a link between inside and outside. I decide which outsider enters. The flux and flow are under my control. The wise blood is either kept or discarded. I either safeguard the developing child or thrust it into an inappropriate environment. Nobody comes or goes except with my permission and decision. I am the beginning of birth. The sun's mark is what I am. Even though I am within reach of your finger, I remain a mystery and a secret. Most men and most women who were born through me live their entire lives without ever looking at me.

I give the Earth my blood. I create clingy, mucus-filled strings for Grandmother Moon. I possess the best hound I create clingy, mucus-filled strings for Grandmother Moon. I possess the best hound's level of sensitivity and the sagest crone's level of wisdom. I am not innocent, and I never have been. Even though darkness is my constant companion and I only have one eye, I am all-seeing. (How odd that Indian women think I have two eyes.)

I am capable of standing my ground against those attempting to storm my portal by being firm and powerful. I am aware of how to be welcoming and open to those who offer hope for the future. I am capable of dissolving into myself and withdrawing, clearing a path, pushing myself to the limit, and opening wide in sweet submission. I beat inside of you. I am the mouth of your womb, your cervix.

What is the cervix?

The cervix is the uterus' neck. It can be felt with the fingertips and extends into the upper part of the vagina, especially when squatting. You can see your cervix well with the aid of a speculum, a mirror, and a flashlight.

The cervix widens during labor, enabling the baby to emerge from the womb and enter the vagina. Furthermore, the cervix opens slightly to help push menstrual blood out of the uterus and allow sperm to fertilize within. I disagree with the medical consensus that the cervix is "insensitive to pain."

A thin layer of cells known as the epithelium covers the cervix. Additionally, there are two types of cells in the epithelium: those that form columns and those that are flat and scaly. The columnar ones are red like our lips and make up the inner surface of the cervix. The squamous cells, which are flat and pink like some skins, make up the outer surface. The squamocolumnar junction, also known as the "transition zone," is where they converge and is one of the most typical sites for cervical cancer.

A healthy, fertile cervix has a lovely round, red mouth, or the os, and is pink in color. *(PBeforepuberty, the cervix is red throughout because pink squamous cells have not yet covered it.)*

An infected, irritated, or abnormally growing cervix typically appears lumpy, bumpy, extremely red, and weepy. (To make the white lesions of HPV visible, a vinegar wash is required.)

The health of the cervix can be impacted by a wide range of microorganisms, such as parasites, bacteria, and viruses, as well as wear and tear from childbirth and sexual activity. Cervicitis, erosion, dysplasia, HPV infections, and cancer comprise the four main classifications of cervical distress, ranked from least to most severe.

Cervicitis: cervix inflammation

- **Acute cervicitis** is an inflammation of the cervix (reddening, swelling, and occasionally bleeding). Cervicitis may occur after a challenging delivery, vacuum aspiration, or trauma. Hormone use, including the use of birth control pills and menopause hormone supplements, as well as irritation from an IUD's string, can cause it. However, most often, a bacterial, viral, or fungal infection like Trichomonas vaginalis, Candida albicans, or Haemophilus vaginalis is what causes cervicitis. Cervicitis can be symptomless or cause discomfort during sexual activity, genital itching and burning, and/or discharge. It is typically successful to use a specific drug or herbal treatment to eliminate infectious organisms.

If irritation and redness persist without an infection, daily application of aloe vera gel, honey, or vitamin E oil for two to three weeks usually works.

- **Chronic cervicitis.** When cervix inflammation and infection persist untreated for a protracted period chronic cervicitis results. Depending on the infection, foul-smelling discharges, sometimes accompanied by pelvic pain, may come and go. The cervix thickens, cysts protrude, and scars and tears from childbirth and gynecological treatments build up. As with using a backhoe to level the ground, orthodox medicine clears the inflamed tissue using antibiotics and surgery; feminism-minded doctors view this as over-treating. Alternative methods, like a meticulous gardener, work to get rid of infections, reverse precancerous changes, and improve the woman's and her cervix's health with the least amount of disruption. Surgery is advised if the condition gets worse or doesn't improve after 3–12 months of treatment.

Cervical Erosion/Eversion

Although they are not the same, even doctors frequently mix them up. Eversion and erosion occur when columnar cells grow too quickly and push the squamous cells aside. In an eversion, the boundaries between the cells are typically distinct. In an erosion, there is no distinct border.

- **Cervical eversions.** Although the columnar cells are spilling out of the os rather than remaining confined to the interior of the cervix, cervical eversions still demonstrate a distinct boundary between the two types of cells. When the hormones that cause cervical eversions, such as birth control pills, are removed, the condition returns to normal.

Some women are born with "congenital" eversion, which regresses until puberty, may be particularly noticeable if she is pregnant, and regresses after menopause. Eversion typically doesn't need treatment; if it's mistaken for erosion, excessive treatment is likely.

- **Cervical erosion.** Any redness on the cervix, from an abrasion to a full-blown infection, is frequently referred to as "cervical erosion." In addition to being incorrect, it is absurd. "[It] conjures up a terrifying image of the cervix wasting away like bare earth after a heavy rain." Conservative medical professionals might advise removing the "eroded" tissue. Cervical erosion can be treated with alternative methods quite successfully; if drugs or surgery are chosen, complementary medicines can lessen side effects and speed up recovery.

Cells in the cervix that are abnormal in cervical dysplasia

Oftentimes, dysplasias regress without treatment. Both traditional and alternative circles frequently engage in overtreatment.

- **Infected with HPV**

Rarely manifesting any symptoms, this silent infection is typically treated by the immune system. Of the sixty varieties that are known, a few can lead to cervical cancer. Cervical cancer is more common in poor women, who are also more likely to be diagnosed with it, die from it, and benefit from required vaccination campaigns.

Unfortunately, the vaccine only protects against HPV before a woman has had any contact with it, whether sexual or otherwise.

- **Breast Cancer**

When the immune system fails to stop abnormal cell growth brought on by HPV, it can invade nearby tissues and even travel through the blood to distant locations. Cervical cancer is fatal if left untreated. Nearly all cases are curable when discovered early.

Your Healthy Cervix

Maintaining the health of your cervix is very similar to maintaining the health of your entire body, with a few exceptions.

If you never looked at or touched your face, just think how challenging it would be to maintain its health. Even though it might seem strange, it's important to examine and touch your cervix at least once in your life, and it's simple.

Although I have done this in groups, you will need a mirror, a flashlight, a plastic speculum, some private time and space, and a reference book. You can position yourself, the mirror, and the flashlight so you can see your cervix with a little wiggling and jiggling. Amazing!

How can one obtain a speculum? The next time you get a gynecological exam, you can ask to keep the one they are currently using. Can you purchase one at the pharmacy?

The uterus includes the cervix, which is made healthier by the same herbs that strengthen and nourish the womb: motherwort tincture and raspberry leaf infusion.

The cervix is exposed to harmful bacteria, viruses, and fungi as part of the vagina, typically from sex but not exclusively. Additionally, when the vagina is traumatized, the cervix also experiences trauma. Maintaining healthy vaginal and gut flora will keep the cervix and vagina healthy, as well as the overall health of the body. I avoid bubble baths, douches, and feminine hygiene sprays because of this, start my days with a cup of plain yogurt, and am extremely picky about what I let near my vagina.

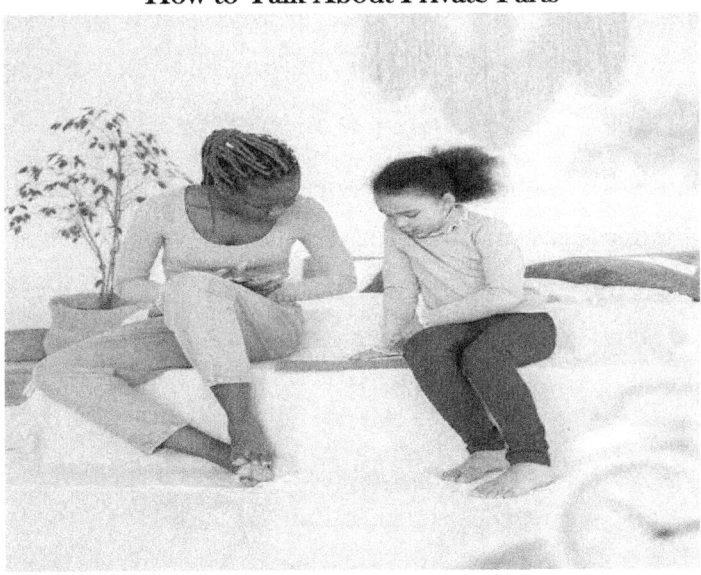

How to Talk About Private Parts

Even though discussing inappropriate touching and private body parts with a child can make any parent feel awkward and uneasy, it's an essential step in ensuring your child's safety. Body-related conversations with your kids should be just as important as any other safety-related discussions. Parental discussions about appropriate and inappropriate touching should take up the same amount of time as other safety preparations. Use these pointers as a guide to help you and your child engage in an informal, interesting, and fun conversation.

When you are prepared to talk with your child, focus solely on them and move at a pace that gives them time to ask questions, air their concerns, and express their thoughts. Children will pick them up whether attitudes are communicated verbally, nonverbally, or through body language and voice tones. Throughout the conversation, it's critical to keep your sense of self and your behavior in check. It's kind of amusing and interesting because it almost feels like you're telling a kid a story.

You must have a positive influence on your child when you speak to him or her to prevent nervousness and body-related anxiety. Being organized and deliberate will aid in conveying the message in an encouragingly conveying the message:

- Use a calm voice;
- Keep the information as simple as possible;
- Have a sense of humor; and, most importantly, be relaxed and sensitive.

This is because young children can easily become embarrassed, perplexed, or reluctant to participate in the conversation.

It's crucial to teach your child the proper anatomical terms during the conversation rather than using nicknames for body parts. Parents frequently refer to various body parts with slang terms, but just as we refer to our ears, noses, and hands, so do we when we discuss our private parts, which include the breasts, penis, and vagina. Knowing the right terms will help your child accurately describe what happened to you, other responsible adults, and perhaps law enforcement if something bad happens to them. Otherwise, the legal system frequently rejects it and doesn't take what they're saying seriously.

When teaching your child about inappropriate touching, keep in mind the importance of clear communication between you and your child. Your child should not feel embarrassed to discuss their body with you in a comfortable setting. He or she should be aware that they have a right to speak up and express themselves when it comes to matters involving their body. The main message of the discussion is that parents must convey to their children that their bodies are something to be proud of, that they own them, and that they should feel at ease with both.

How to Care for Private Parts

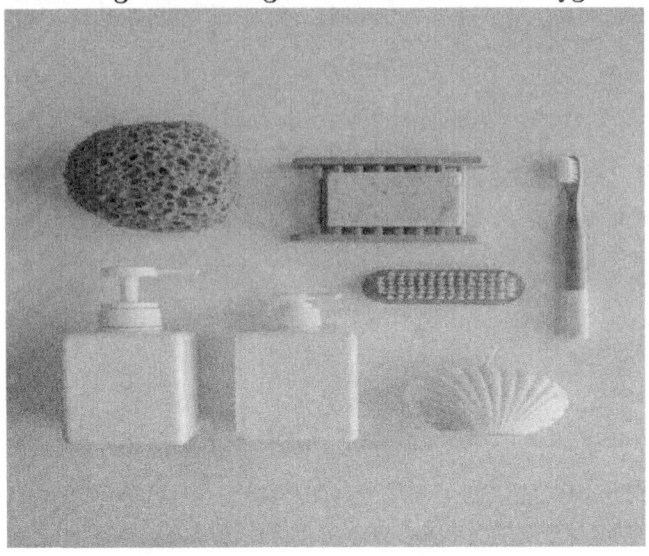

Teaching Your Daughter about Personal Hygiene

Even though it might seem awkward and unnecessary, it's important to start talking to your daughter about vaginal care when she's young. It's not necessary to get into specifics right away, but using and teaching your daughter the proper terms for her body parts, such as "vagina" and "vulva," as well as briefly explaining how her body functions, is a great place to start.

Women's bodies are oversexualized in our culture, and girls and women are made to feel as though their bodies are for other people's approval. It's crucial to remind your daughter that her body belongs to her and no one else when you talk to her about touching and what her body's boundaries are.

Teach your daughter to always wipe her vagina from the front to the back when it comes to teaching personal hygiene to prevent infection. Give her a gentle cleanser, like our feminine wash, to use to clean her vagina, and teach her that she should never use a washcloth that could potentially contain bacteria. Outside of mainstream advertising, vaginas don't smell like flowers, and a typical odor or discharge is perfectly normal. Tell her that while her vagina isn't "dirty," if it ever itches or burns, that could be a sign of a medical problem, and she should let you know.

Even before she reaches puberty, there is no reason why your daughter shouldn't be aware of menstruation. It's a normal aspect of womanhood and nothing to be afraid of. To provide your daughter with a foundational understanding of menstrual products, learn how to talk to her about her period. In this manner, your daughter will grow up feeling secure and knowing that these physical changes are natural.

When you take the time to talk to your daughter about her incredible body as she goes through different stages of life, you can make sure that she will continue to have a healthy sense of self-worth as she gets older and understands the power that she and her vagina have! Having a healthy conversation with your daughter about her body can strengthen your relationship.

Teaching Your Daughter about the Importance of Wearing Clean Underwear

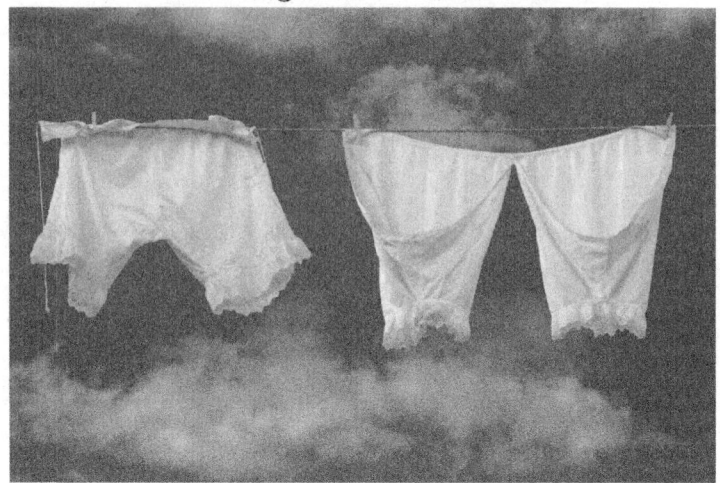

1. Explain to your daughter that wearing clean underwear is important because it helps keep her skin healthy and free of bacteria that can cause irritation and infection. It also helps to keep her feeling comfortable and confident in all her outfits.
2. Talk about the consequences of not wearing clean underwear. Explain to your daughter that if she doesn't wear clean underwear, she could get skin rashes, infections, and odors. It can also make her uncomfortable and embarrassed if she has to take off her clothes for any reason.
3. Let her know that wearing clean underwear is a sign of good hygiene. Explain to your daughter that taking good care of her body includes wearing clean underwear every day. This is a sign that she takes pride in her appearance and respects herself.

4. Show her how to clean her underwear properly. Explain to your daughter that she should always wash her underwear after each wear. She should also make sure to separate her whites from her colors and use the appropriate temperature settings for washing and drying.
5. Encourage her to have enough clean underwear. Explain to your daughter that it is important to have enough pairs of clean underwear so she doesn't have to constantly do laundry. Having enough pairs of clean underwear will also help her feel more comfortable and confident.

Teaching Your Daughter about the Dangers of Abusing Her Private Parts

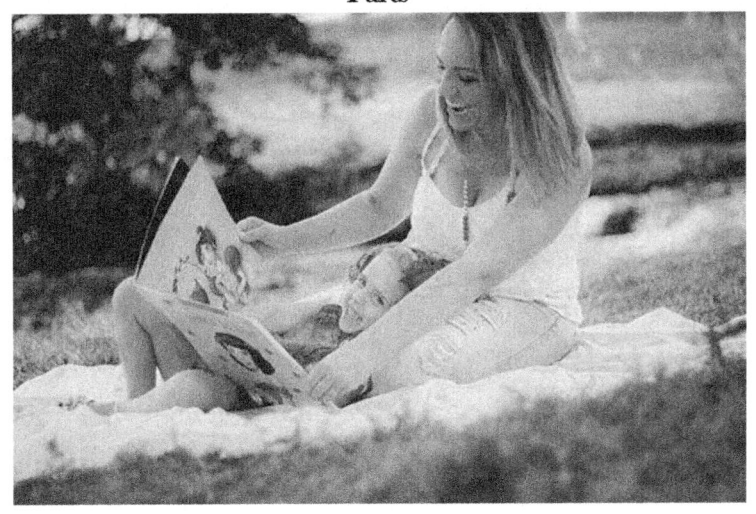

Teaching your daughter about the dangers of abusing her private parts is an important part of ensuring her safety and well-being. Too often, this sensitive topic is left out of conversations, leaving your daughter vulnerable to potential harm. But by providing her with the knowledge and understanding she needs, you can help her stay safe and prevent potential abuse.

Start by talking to your daughter about her body and the different parts of it. Explain to her the correct words for her private parts and that they are special and should only be touched by her or with her permission. Emphasize that it's important to be careful with her private parts and that she should always tell you if anyone touches her there.

Model the kind of language you want her to use when discussing private parts. Avoid using slang, nicknames, or anything else that could make her feel uncomfortable or embarrassed. Make sure she knows that it is OK to talk to you about her body and private parts and that she will never get in trouble for doing so.

Educate your daughter about whom she can and can't trust when it comes to her body. Remind her that no one should ever ask her to keep secrets about her private parts and that she should always tell an adult if she feels unsafe.

Reassure her that it is not her fault if someone abuses her private parts. Explain that it is always the abuser's fault and that she should never feel ashamed or embarrassed if something like this happens.

Finally, be sure to emphasize that if something ever happens to her, she should tell you right away. Reassure her that you will always believe in her, support her, and do whatever it takes to keep her safe.

By teaching your daughter about the dangers of abusing her private parts, you are taking a proactive step to ensure her safety and well-being. Not only will she know how to protect herself, but you can also help create a safe environment in which she can feel comfortable discussing these important topics.

Chapter Three
Sexting and Sex Education

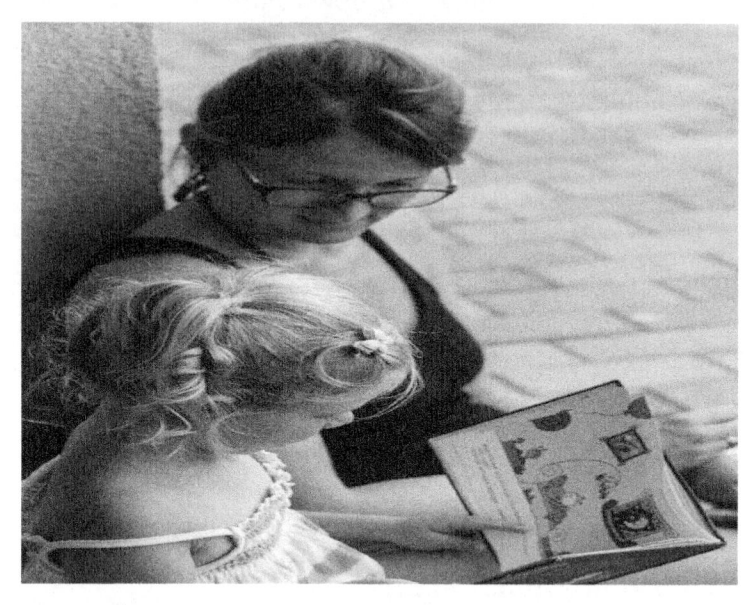

Sex and sexual innuendo are prevalent in our culture today, with sex and sexual innuendo appearing in a variety of media, including music, movies, television shows, and advertisements. Recently, even Obama couldn't help but declare that insulation is "sexy."

There are no longer any secrets; everything is public, and our kids have joined in the trend with a worrying one of their own. Sending sexually explicit electronic messages or images is known as "sexting," and most parents are unaware of the emotional, psychological, and social repercussions of sexting in addition to what their children are posting online or on their mobile devices.

Parents must be involved in the education of children about the dangers of [sexting] and ensure that they are keeping an eye on how their offspring use their computers and cell phones.

Teenagers today depend heavily on technology, so they must learn how to use it safely, wisely, and morally. Giving them the knowledge and judgment they require is the responsibility of parents and teachers.

The majority of the schools in our country run ongoing campaigns to educate students about sexting risks, cyberbullying, and internet safety. These special presentations are typically given to students during the school day and to parents and the general public during the evening.

However, as previously stated, in addition to what schools can do, parents have a responsibility to watch over their children and educate them about the dangers of sexting and other types of cell phones and Internet misuse.

I taught you how to cross the street; the parents need to sit down and tell their children. I'll show you how to stay secure online.

So whether you believe your child is sexting or not, have that repeated, nonjudgmental conversation.

- Start by learning what she believes or knows about sexting.
- Find out if she or any of her friends have ever sent or received incendiary images or messages, whether through email or text.

- Check her Facebook, MySpace, and cell phone frequently to see whom she communicates with.
- Ask him to leave his cell phone on the kitchen counter whenever he is home and put the computer in a well-traveled area of the house.
- Establish usage restrictions by deciding on a reasonable number of texts and photos that can be sent. If she crosses the line, either deny her access to her computer and phone for a predetermined period or severely curtail her texting allowance.
- Describe to her the importance of reporting any offensive messages or images to you so that you can take note of who sent them, what they were, and the sender's contact information.
- Remind her that sent messages rarely remain private once they have been sent, even to just one person, and that they frequently circulate for a very long time and in front of the entire world.
- Discuss with her articles about actual situations in which children were discovered, suspended, expelled, or even charged with child pornography (a felony) and threatened with being listed as sex offenders.
- Describe the emotional toll that children's photos can take on them, sometimes leading to suicide as in the case of a young Florida woman, and explain why you are so concerned.

In other words, exercise caution and maintain open lines of communication. Although our children are technologically savvy, they are also naive and occasionally too trusting. They need to understand that we're fairly astute ourselves and are aware of the dangers they run when they act like the adolescents they are and make poor decisions.

How to Have a Sexual Conversation with Your Girl

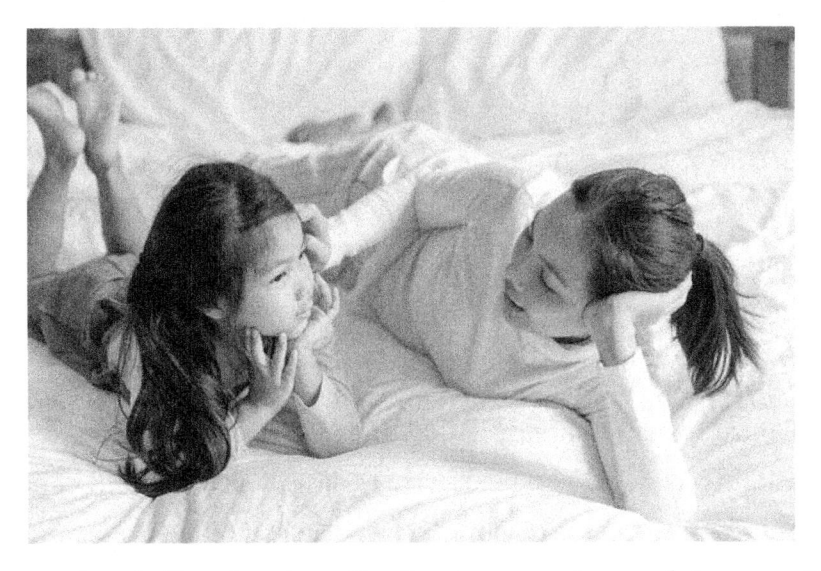

It can be challenging to talk about sex and sexual issues with teenagers, especially parents. Society's perceptions have changed as a result of how sex and sexuality are portrayed in the media, and there is now a much greater openness than there was when I was a young woman. When my daughter was getting ready to start middle school, I thought we should have a conversation about the repercussions and dangers of sex. My daughter had already told me about a friend of hers who was fourteen years old and pregnant, as well as a thirteen-year-old classmate who had already experienced two STDs. This final bit of knowledge was gleaned from the sex education curriculum the school district used in the sixth grade for students whose parents gave their child permission to enroll in the class as part of "health."

It is crucial to start and maintain a conversation between parents and their children because, regardless of their chronological age, most teenagers are developing and maturing emotionally somewhere between adolescence and adulthood. Serious conversations must be handled with care, especially those involving peers or social-emotional issues. The key is to avoid alienating teenagers by undervaluing their knowledge or experience, to be informal rather than demanding, to avoid lecturing, and to involve them in the conversation. Whatever the subject of the conversation with their children, parents need to listen as well as talk.

I conducted research on the Internet and at the neighborhood public library to make sure I was knowledgeable and capable of taking on this task. I obtained this information from the county health department and the Planned Parenthood affiliate in my area. The Kansas Kids Count book provided me with statistics on teen pregnancy, single parents, and other information. Every state gathers statistical information by township, county, and city and makes it available in some form of written source. I was prepared to try and talk to my daughter at that point, hoping she wouldn't be too embarrassed to engage in conversation with her "mother."

I waited until my then ten-year-old son's Boy Scout troop was out camping before I sent him. My husband was at work and worked the second shift. I brought up the subject of boys while watching a television movie with my daughter, asking if she had a boyfriend. I was well aware that parents frequently find out about their child's first boyfriend after the fact. Even though my daughter did not yet have a boyfriend, she added that she did not want a boyfriend because men only wanted sex, whether it be oral sex or physical copulation, and demanded that the girl give up all of her friends. They also did not want the girl to have any other regular male friends. She had discovered this from a close friend who had confided in my daughter when she needed someone to talk to about her first boyfriend and how she was handling it.

I had been waiting for an opening, and here it was. I first explained to my daughter that I wasn't trying to imply that she had engaged in intense touching or sex or that I was trying to lecture her; rather, I just wanted to make sure she had the resources and knowledge she would need if she ever felt physically or emotionally attracted to a guy. I told her that since my intention was not to lecture or exert pressure on her, she should jump in and correct me if she thought I was mistaken or misinformed about anything, let me know if I was making her uncomfortable, and share any information she might have. I discussed the lengths to which many boys would go to initiate physical contact with a girl, including telling her that he loved her and would never cheat on her and that if she loved him, she would have sex with him, or threatening to end the relationship if she refused to consent to his advances. My daughter continued, saying that one of her friends had also gone through the ordeal of having a man tell his male classmates and friends at school that they had engaged in "oral sex," even though no such act had occurred.

This then sparked a conversation about how a girl might react in a comparable circumstance. I said that this lie had to be very painful for the other girl, and I felt for what she was going through. I also mentioned how many young men enjoy boasting about their victories, whether explicit or implicit, to persuade their peers of their prowess in the bedroom. We discussed some possible actions my daughter's friend could take, such as ignoring the man and any of his friends who might make advances or crude remarks, expressing regret that the man must lie to feel important, or simply refusing to respond to his lie.

My daughter replied that if it happened to her, she'd sarcastically say to the guy, "Maybe in your dreams," in front of his friends. This was a good illustration of adolescent brilliance, which would serve my daughter and other adolescents well. I concurred that embarrassing a young man might be effective. I was able to add a wealth of information by having a mutual and open dialogue from the start. My daughter made some brief comments and posed some thoughtful inquiries.

I once emphasized to my daughter that I wanted her to wait until she was married and that I did not support having sex before getting married. I added that my main objective was to prepare her for that eventuality and that I was aware that I would have no control over any decision she would ultimately make regarding any sexual activity or when she chose to become sexually active. We discussed various STDs and their symptoms, even though the local children had already learned some of that information during sex education.

Because the male did not want to wear a prophylactic, my daughter brought up the topic of peers who took alternative precautions to prevent an unwanted pregnancy. Then, I was able to inform her that the sexual "myths" that many teenagers who lack knowledge hold to be true are wholly untrue. These myths included the notion that using the rhythm method, having the young man remove himself from the woman before ejaculating, determining the timing of the fertile portion of the girl's cycle using body temperature, etc., would significantly reduce the likelihood of unintended pregnancy.

I was asked if having oral sex was considered sex in and of itself. My response was that, while it was true that this was a sexual act intended to prevent the guy from having a girl become pregnant, it was disrespectful to the girl and demeaning to her. Depending on how promiscuous both parties had been in the past, the girl and the guy could still contract STDs like herpes, chlamydia, and AIDS. I discovered that many of my daughter's peers were engaging in oral sex as a means of "pleasuring their boyfriends and not getting pregnant" during the discussion of oral sex.

I discussed the various types of love with my daughter and later with my son, including infatuation, hormonal lust, non-sexual love for someone of the opposite sex, and the profound emotional love that results from adult emotional maturity. I explained that if a relationship is based primarily on sex, it is very unlikely to last for very long at any age. This is also one of the main reasons that many relationships end in divorce court, or separation and abandonment if the couple is not married.

Last but not least, I advised my daughter to carefully weigh the pros and cons of any future sexual decisions she made, use protection to prevent STDs, and combine the use of a prophylactic with a foam or other contraceptive because a prophylactic can be damaged.

She would never tell me she was going to have sex, I added, but I would let her half-sister, who was then 16 years old, know she had my permission to assist her in obtaining birth control at that time. I did mention that the only way to ensure she wouldn't contract an STD or become pregnant is through abstinence.

Only a small percentage of teenagers will inform their parents of their plans to engage in sexual activity. The parent-child relationship and parental nurturing, which are very important to a teenager even though they might not express it out loud, could be jeopardized by that because it would be too intrusive and "not cool." Additionally, it's a knowledge that most parents, including myself, don't want to have. But at least I was confident that I had prepared my daughter for the majority of scenarios and that she would ultimately make the decision.

Educating Your Girl about the Value of Modesty

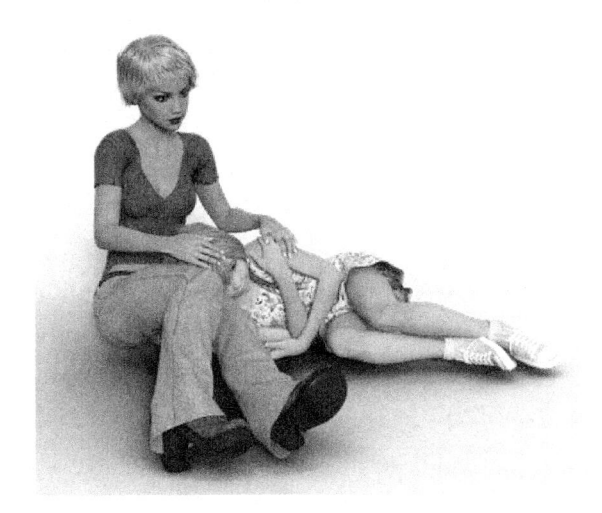

Seeing girls and women constantly exposed to immoral and immodest images and behaviors is upsetting and demoralizing. This devaluation of women's worth starts shockingly early in life. In addition to teaching boys a lack of respect for women, this makes young girls believe they must look a certain way to be accepted and liked.

The task of instilling in their children the value of modesty and virtue can at times seem overwhelming and perhaps even impossible. Parents can, however, teach their children to respect themselves and others through their appearance and behavior if they are persistent and patient with them. Your girls will become happier, more self-assured women who demand respect as a result of this.

It's never too early to emphasize how important appropriate attire is. You might believe that your little girl shouldn't care what she wears because she doesn't have hips or breasts. But keep in mind that she only has this body shape right now. She's going to be a young woman before you know it. If those values were taught to her as a child, it will be much simpler for her to comprehend and appreciate modest dress. Your daughter will continue to understand and value the significance of dressing appropriately as she grows and matures if you set the example for her at a young age.

Parents should set a good example. Bear in mind that your daughter has grown up watching you. She looks up to you and looks to you to set the example for her actions and behaviors, even though you may not be aware of it. This also applies to your attire. You are establishing a standard for her future wardrobe by demonstrating to her that you value your body by dressing appropriately.

Teach your kid to take the initiative rather than follow. Her friends and acquaintances will undoubtedly be dressed in the newest trends, including some scantily clad outfits, but she is under no obligation to follow suit. Help her forge her path and establish her fashion trends so she won't have to rely on her friends for style inspiration. She will feel more confident in her decisions as a result. Her independent demeanor will gain the respect of those around her and assist her in avoiding perilous pitfalls, such as those involving sexual compromise.

Keep an eye on what your daughter does, listens to, and watches, and assist her in avoiding inappropriate content. The media wants every young girl to believe that to be a real princess, she must dress revealingly, purchase the most expensive name brands, and engage in worldly and immoral activities. However, you can demonstrate to your daughters that adopting moral, useful, and admirable behaviors will bring them true happiness. Your young child will have a better attitude about herself and her role in the world as a strong and confident woman if they stay away from music, movies, and peer groups that denigrate motherhood and womanhood.

When it comes to teaching girls the importance of respecting themselves, their bodies, and their self-worth, parents have their work cut out for them. They've been inundated with messages from the outside world that make it seem like living frugally, modestly, and virtuously is outdated, if not outright unacceptable. However, it is ultimately the job of the parents to impart to their children the moral and ethical ideals that will allow them to feel the joy that comes from respecting themselves and the world around them.

Protecting Your Girl from Sexual Predators

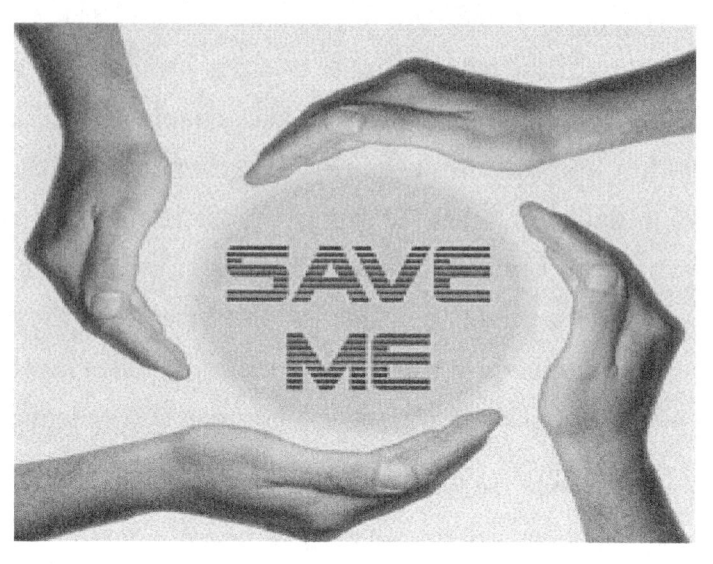

As a new mother, I researched breastfeeding, choking hazards, and vaccines. However, I had no idea when to talk to my daughter about potential child sexual abuse or what to say. Given that I work in the field of child sexual abuse, this was especially shocking. When my daughter was almost three, I had been a prosecutor of child abuse and sex crimes for ten years. Since children cannot always tell if they have been touched, it was crucial to have an early discussion about what constitutes a good touch and a bad touch. I knew this from my experience at work. My pediatrician worked for a large practice with a website that offered helpful advice on healthy eating and effective parenting. I started my search for an answer on his website. I looked through the website, but I couldn't find anything that even hinted at the topic. I waited until my daughter's next scheduled doctor's appointment before addressing the doctor directly. He advised me to talk to her about these things as soon as she is old enough to be left alone and has rudimentary communication skills. He instructed you to inform her that the areas of her body hidden by her bathing suit are private and should not be touched. I inquired as to why this was not mentioned on the company website. "I don't know, taboo?" He shrugged his shoulders.

Once she was old enough to leave my sight, which is right now, but without more direction, I couldn't have this discussion. What if I make a mistake? Suppose I frightened her. I went to the nation's largest children's library here in New York City and asked the librarian for all of the books on discussing good touch and bad touch with kids. Five minutes later, the woman reappeared carrying a stack of books on the sense of touch, including ones on how to touch both hard and soft objects. The librarian didn't get what I was saying. I tried it again. I explained to her that I wanted to talk to my three-year-old about the fact that nobody should touch her intimate areas. The librarian's face lit up in recognition, and this time she came back bearing several books on the subject I had requested. Though the majority of them were written in the 1990s, the most recent was only five years old. They were all written at a reading level and with an attention span appropriate for sixth graders, I discovered after reading through each one. They were undoubtedly much too complex for my son, who will turn three in a few months.

I reflected on why a book like the one I was looking for was as crucial as I became frustrated by the scarcity of age-appropriate reading materials. I thought of a trial I had handled years ago that had made a big impression on me. I brought charges against a stepfather who had been sexually abusing a nine-year-old girl since she was six. She kept it secret. The girl once caught a segment of "The Oprah Winfrey Show" about young victims of physical abuse. The "Tortured Children" episode empowered the girl by conveying the straightforward advice, "If you're being abused, tell your parents." Go to school and tell your teacher if you are unable to tell your parents. The following day, the girl went to school and informed her teacher after receiving the message. Her teacher informed the principal, who then got in touch with Child Services, who alerted the police. The defendant was found guilty and is currently serving a protracted prison sentence after I prosecuted the case on behalf of the District Attorney's office.

I have frequently recalled that wonderful, brave nine-year-old girl. I realized that all it took to put an end to her nightmare after three excruciating years was a TV program urging her to "tell a teacher." If only there were a way to spread that message further so that kids everywhere could hear it, I mused.

The prevention of child sexual abuse is the focus of numerous organizations. One of the first services for battered women and sexual assault victims in the Midwest was provided by the Rape and Abuse Crisis Center of Fargo-Moorhead. Children who have experienced sexual abuse can receive both individual and group counseling services for battered women and sexual assault victims in the Midwest provided by the Rape and Abuse Crisis Center of

Fargo-Moorhead. Children who have experienced sexual abuse can receive both individual and group counseling. They provide invaluable assistance to the families of victims, but they also engage in outreach to stop abuse from happening. Their Red Flag Green Flag Sexual Abuse Prevention Program goes above and beyond the fundamentals of teaching personal safety to children in elementary school.

Children should learn early on that their bodies are private. Education is unquestionably the key to prevention, and parents should take advantage of any teachable moment to speak with their children.

Parents must be aware of some fundamental facts regarding their child's sexuality. The first reality is that all children can be victims of sexual abuse. It doesn't care if you're white, black, Hispanic, wealthy, or follow a particular religion. Unfortunately, it occurs everywhere.

The second reality is that most kids do not report being sexually abused. When a child is the victim of child sexual abuse, they frequently experience confusion, shame, guilt, fear of not being believed, and orders not to tell anyone, unlike a child who runs to Mommy when he falls and scrapes his knee.

The third sad reality is that parents do not discuss child sexual abuse with their kids or how to prevent it. Unfortunately, even good parents I know rarely discuss their children's bodies with them. They are not being silent out of apathy; rather, they are being silent because, like me, they are unsure of what to say, when to say it, or how to say it. Parents frequently avoid the conversation because they mistakenly think that neither they nor their family will ever experience sexual abuse. Sadly, all reliable statistics point to the opposite. According to studies, 1 in 3 girls and 1 in 6 boys will experience molestation, and many of them will suffer the incapacitating effects of this behavior into adulthood.

The good news is that parents can take action to change these alarming statistics and they can start a conversation with their kids.

She teaches kids the difference between good touches (also known as "green flag" touches) and bad touches in an age-appropriate and non-threatening way as early as preschool ("red flag" touches). Children are taught what to do if they come across someone who exhibits a "red flag" touch.

Say no, leave, and then inform a helper

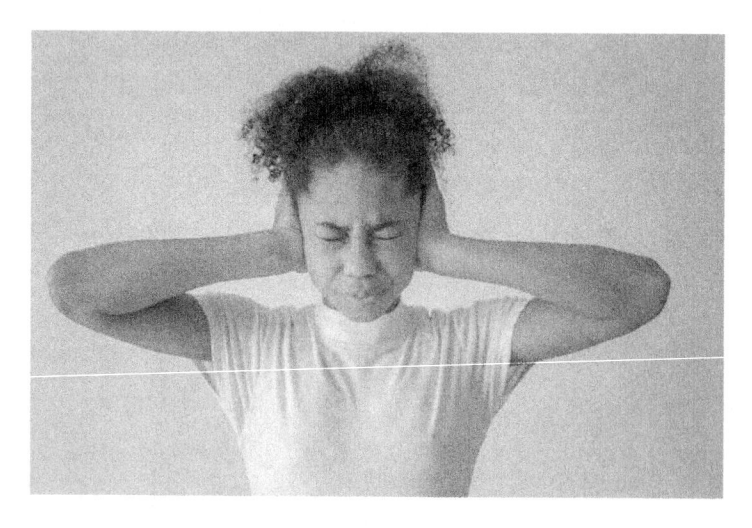

Most frequently, the child's abuser is someone they know. It might be a friend, a stepfather, an older sibling, a cousin, a babysitter, a coach, etc. Naturally, this makes sense because those we trust to be alone with our child would have the chance to do something that needs a certain amount of privacy. It makes sense to wonder: What is typical indications of abuse? What should I do if I suspect anything abusive? How can I assist my child in recovering from the trauma of abuse? Parents who are concerned about their children can find information at the Rape and Crisis Center. There is currently a war in progress. Child predators have figured out how to approach our kids. They are aware of the preferences, needs, and wants of our kids. The children do not disclose the abuse because they know what to say. This should serve as a wake-up call to all parents who do not discuss the prevention of child sexual abuse. We are leaving our kids out there naked by delaying having this conversation with them. We are capable of winning this war. Engage the youth in your life in conversation because every young child should be taught that their bodies are private. The best gift you could give them is this.

Chapter Four

Good Touch. Bad Touch. What They Are All About?

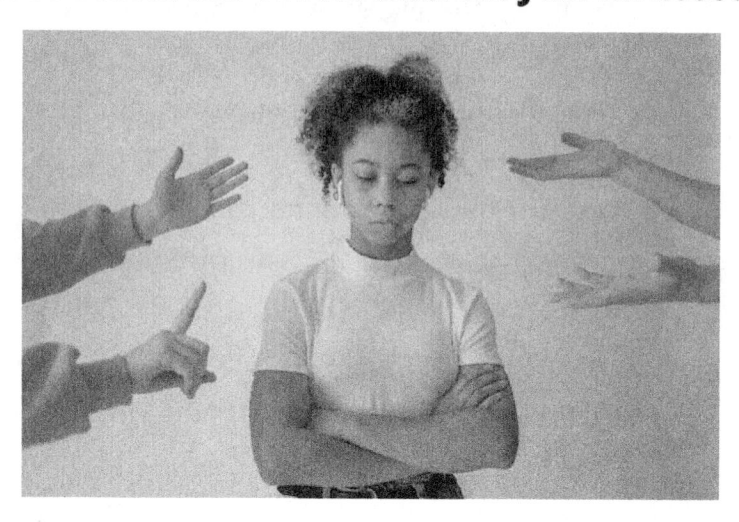

She informed her kids that a familiar relative would be dropping by on that particular day. Everyone was content, excluding Katrina. The mother stared intently into her daughter's eyes, unable to tell whether her daughter was feeling fear, sadness, or anger. Katrina was going through all of them at once. What is it, her mother inquired, puzzled. You keep that expression on your face whenever he visits you. When will you start showing others respect and courtesy? Nothing happened; the child simply continued to watch television.

After an hour had passed, Katrina was circling her mother, attempting to talk to her despite her fear. Although the mother should have noticed her child's expression and need for communication, she was preoccupied with getting the house ready for guests. She didn't realize it until Katrina broke down in a severe crying fit and begged her mother to let her stay in her room while they were around. To overcome her confusion and rage, Katrina's mother gently leads her daughter to the adjacent room and inquires, "What bothers you so much about this relative?" "I used to dread his touches, even though they seemed normal, like when he touched my hands," Katrina said in response. Later, even though it seemed normal, he started touching other parts of my body, like my shoulders, and it bothered me. He attempted to touch my body in private places during his previous visit.

Katrina's story is the story shared by many children. There are two dimensions to it. First, parents need to close attention to how they handle their kids' fears and other feelings toward other people. How parents can comprehend and evaluate the situation without getting emotionally upset would be covered in a separate book. The second is the significance of teaching kids how to recognize various kinds of touches and how to respond to each, which is the subject of this chapter.

Children frequently experience various people's touching. Sometimes those touches are tender ones, like the ones their parents give them. Other touches, like those they experience at home or school, are routine. A child may experience professional touches occasionally, such as those at the doctor's office, and accidental or random touches more frequently, such as those he might experience while playing with friends or being around them. A child's reactions to most of these touches can range from comfort to indifference because they are an ordinary part of his life. Such touches are referred to as "good touches" because they do not cause confusion or harm to children.

Some touches exactly resemble "good touches." However, their fundamental differences are striking. Such touches are referred to as "bad touches" because they cause a child to feel distressed, harmed, and overwhelmed with the urge to flee.

Many young children can tell the difference between a "good touch" and a "bad touch" without thinking about it. The child's confidence in his instincts grows along with this ability. Although being able to distinguish between different touches is crucial, a child cannot be protected unless he also has two other abilities. The first would be the capacity to respond, and the second would be the capacity to interact with an adult (a parent, for example) to seek safety and find solutions.

When children want to move forward after realizing they have experienced a "bad touch," they frequently face significant obstacles. A child who hasn't been taught how to behave appropriately in these circumstances might feel overpowered by feelings of uncertainty and fear. He might not act in a way that is best for him or that is safe for him. Additionally, he might have trouble telling his parents, for example, what he went through and how he feels. The child may fear that his parents won't believe him or take him seriously if the abuser is someone close to the family, which is typically the case. The child is always the main and most unfortunate party because he is not provided with the safety measures he needs.

Children's protection depends on two main factors for the duration of their lives. First, they should have more confidence in their instincts and be taught basic, useful manners without using horror or fear as a teaching tool. The second would be to ensure that they and their parents or other caregivers always have an open line of communication marked by love, tolerance, attentive listening, and sympathy. This is done to foster an environment where kids can express their fears without fear of retaliation. Additionally, it contributes to the development of an atmosphere free from concerns about being dismissed or mistrusted. It should be noted that a child's claim that he experienced a "bad touch" does not necessarily imply that the other person is meant to be abusive. It does, however, imply that the child is bothered by something that is significant and necessitates immediate and serious care.

Chapter Five

Puberty Problems While Growing up

Acne during Puberty

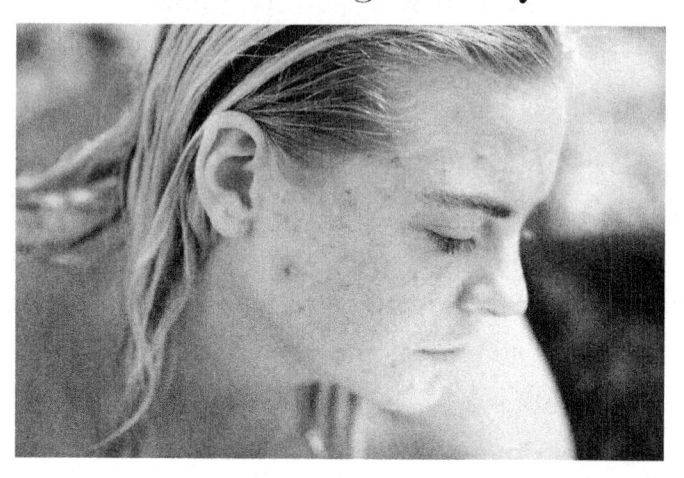

Girls go through a lot of changes during puberty, both physical and psychological. Menstruation, body composition, body and facial hair growth, growth spurts, skin changes, and body odor are a few of these modifications. As the amount of fat tissue in the breasts, hips, and thighs grows during puberty, the body undergoes physical changes that result in the typical female shape. What impact does acne have on girls during this challenging and emotional time, given all the changes that occur during puberty?

Girls who have acne may feel more physically and emotionally stressed during puberty. Due to the increased oil secretions in the skin, two of the numerous changes in girls during puberty include the severity and propensity of acne. Girls going through puberty may also feel low self-esteem, experience mood swings, and become more irritable. When puberty begins, even girls who have always been confident can experience low self-esteem.

If a girl also has acne, these changes during puberty may be more pronounced. There are actions you can take to lessen acne issues, which may support girls during this trying time.

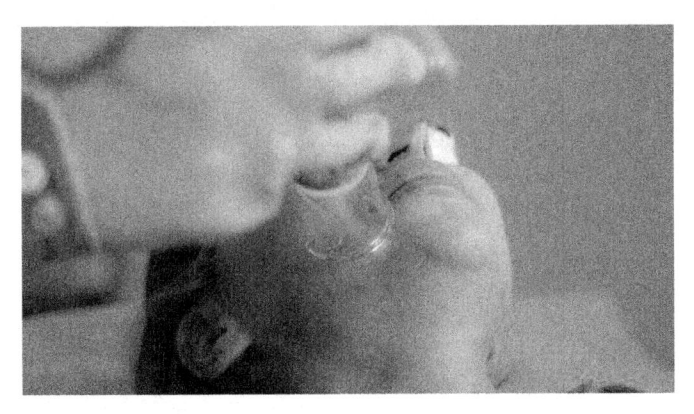

Girls' Practical Acne Treatments

The first step in treating acne is proper skin care. There are many skin care items available on the market that could treat acne. The first thing to do is gently wash your face twice daily. Choose a cleanser with salicylic acid, benzoyl peroxide, or sulfur because these ingredients kill the bacteria that cause acne. Avoid washing your face too frequently or using abrasive cleansers on your face because gentle cleansing is crucial.

When attempting to control acne, it's important to use non-comedogenic products. Non-comedogenic is less likely to clog skin pores, cause acne, or cause blackheads. There are many non-comedogenic goods on the market, including lipsticks, moisturizers, makeup that treats acne, and even makeup.

If acne cannot be controlled by over-the-counter medications, it is a good idea to see a dermatologist who can prescribe the best treatment.

Along with all the other changes that occur in girls during puberty, acne can be physically and mentally taxing. One need not be discouraged because there are numerous treatments for acne available today. Another obstacle that young women must overcome is the appearance of acne during puberty.

Teen anxiety and the puberty blues: a nightmare for parents

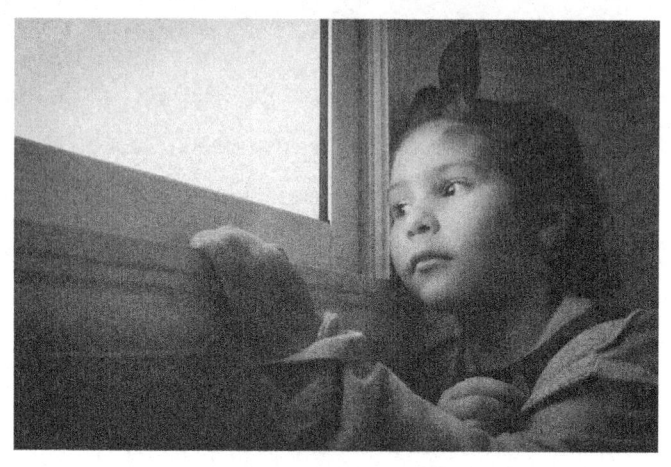

Has your adolescent stopped paying attention to you?

Teenage anxiety is frequently the first sign of the onset of puberty. Has your adorable toddler or brash young boy has grown up and stopped taking your advice? Are they growing more obstinate? Have they begun to respond? Do they defy your orders and act irrationally furious when you don't give them what they want?

These are just the typical changes that children go through as they approach puberty, so don't blame the child for them. You will hear from many other parents, and most of the time they will be accurate. Because as children approach puberty, their developing bodies begin to produce the hormones testosterone in boys and estrogen and progesterone in girls, and it is usually these hormones that lead to the physical and emotional changes in children that are challenging for parents to handle.

Your curiosity and comprehension frequently result in miraculous outcomes.

It doesn't help to put the blame on kids or make stricter demands on them to stop their rebellious behavior because kids don't consciously understand what is happening to them as they enter adolescence.

Instead, by empathizing with what they're going through and spending more time with them, talking about their interests (such as the music they're listening to, how their friends are doing, sports with boys, fashion with girls, and, if appropriate, sharing some of your own childhood experiences when you were their age) can frequently lead to miraculous results.

It's time to take a closer look and see if your child's behavior matches any of the alarming anxiety symptoms that kids with anxiety disorders display, especially if your child's behavior becomes more extreme, even outlandish and disturbing, to the point where you start to worry they'll do something reckless or regretful.

Is your adolescent exhibiting signs of anxiety and panic attacks?

Teenagers, unfortunately, experience anxiety and panic attack more frequently than most people realize, and because they often find it difficult to express their deeper emotions, parents frequently attribute their children's unsettling behavior to things like puberty, school, and peer pressure, completely omitting the fact that their child may be dealing with an anxiety or panic disorder.

If a child's anxiety symptoms are disregarded and they are left untreated throughout adolescence, their anxiety-driven fear will not only intensify but will frequently worsen to the point where their behavior spirals out of control and they turn to drugs and alcohol. They will then carry these addictions, along with their anxiety, into adulthood.

"Puberty Blues" is frequently a difficult journey for parents

It's uncommon to find a parent who doesn't love and care for their child, but when facing the difficulties of puberty with their adolescent children, parents frequently discover they need assistance. I was living in New York and earning a living as a television actor when, for the first time, I was cast in my first theatrical stage production and was forced to acknowledge that I had a serious disorder after experiencing anxiety and panic attacks throughout my teens and into my early 20s. In the past, when the pressure got too much, I would treat my anxiety by abusing alcohol and prescription medications. However, being required to perform each night in front of a live audience, I knew it was time to look for treatment at that point. I was finally able to identify my disorder and start to comprehend the cause after talking to numerous people and learning how common the condition was.

Autism Spectrum Disorders

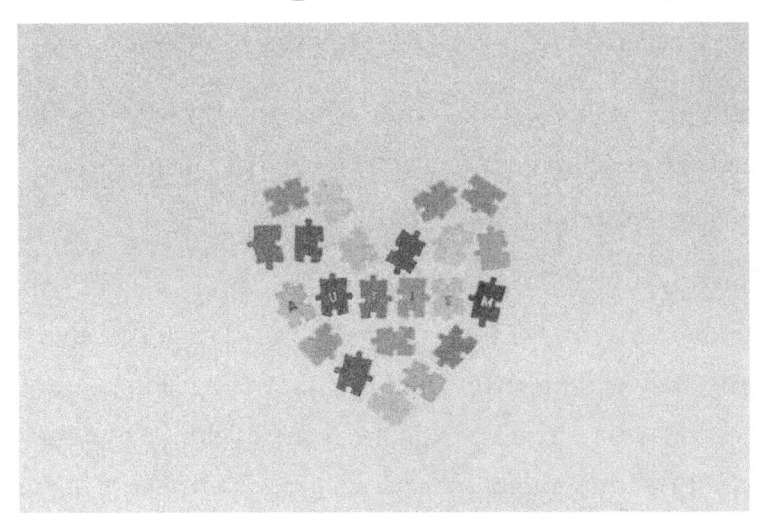

Puberty can be a very delicate and difficult time for a family, even without autism. But when autism is involved, things can get very complicated. Many parents are afraid and nervous about this time in their child's life. You should, however, make an effort to approach this time in a very positive and developmentally focused manner.

Whether or not a person is autistic, sexuality and sex education are significant aspects of life for anyone going through puberty. After all, kids and teenagers are sexual beings. You must impart appropriate sexual expressions and promote healthy attitudes toward sexuality to respect your autistic child's dignity. It will be your responsibility as a parent to keep your child safe.

Many parents worry that their autistic children will regress during adolescence.

A recent study showed that, among the 108 individuals who experienced a noticeable regression during adolescence, half had fully recovered by the time they reached adulthood.

Additionally, the same study supported earlier findings that language development and a better quality of life, in general, are positively correlated with childhood IQ levels.

Consequently, it is reasonable to assume that a child with autism will be able to learn to manage the difficulties and changes associated with puberty. The important thing is to be aware of any questions or ambiguities that he or she might have so that you can assist in settling them. You can incorporate teaching opportunities into your daily activities to help your child learn and rediscover the processes that take place inside their bodies.

Your child's pediatrician might be able to recommend some methods and resources to make the transition to puberty easier for your family and your autistic child. Various books (like "Asperger's Syndrome and Sexuality: From Adolescence Through Adulthood"), pamphlets, websites, and even additional therapies, such as hormone treatments for girls to control menstrual cycles and lessen any discomfort, may fall under this category. This will make a girl's period more predictable so that she will know exactly what day it will start and roughly when it will end. Additionally, each month at the same time of the cycle, the same physical sensations will take place. A careful discussion with your doctor or your child's pediatrician is essential because this course of treatment may be viewed as somewhat controversial.

A psychologist or child psychologist might also be able to give you additional insight into how to help your child transition through puberty as painlessly as possible.

You will be better prepared to handle many questions your child may have, as well as any new transient or long-term symptoms your child may develop, with the help of both a doctor and a psychiatrist.

The Connection: Thyroid Problems and Puberty

One of the primary hormones that regulate the body's metabolism is the thyroid hormone, which is released by the thyroid gland, which is situated just below the neck area. This gland is visible as a small tissue clump close to the throat. By running their hands over the throat region, many people can feel these very finely; however, for some people, they are very noticeable even from a distance as a protruding area under the throat.

Thyroxin, an enzyme, aids in the secretion of the thyroid hormone. Thyroxin is a biochemical substance that helps to absorb iodine from the blood, which speeds up the secretion of thyroid hormone. Iodine is a crucial mineral that is typically present in many kinds of seafood and iodized salts. They are crucial for activating the thyroid gland. Iodine, in other words, is a microelement that the body needs at optimal levels to accelerate the metabolism of the biochemical reaction, but at very low levels. While excessive secretion causes hyperthyroidism, a lack of iodine can cause hypothyroidism.

The majority of girls may experience thyroid issues during puberty.

Although this is a natural occurrence, the disturbances only last a very brief time, possibly up to the first or second menstrual cycle. There may be some irregularities in growth and appearance. You shouldn't be concerned about them. In some extreme situations, thyroid secretion may be lower than the necessary optimal levels or at higher limits. Multiple psychological disturbances, including depression or any change in emotional feelings, loss of appetite, or a feeling of mental weakness, can be brought on by this. These could appear alongside the other typical thyroid imbalance symptoms, such as hair loss, dry skin, etc. By including iodine-rich foods in the diet, these can be easily resolved.

When talking about the effects of thyroid small-cell dysfunction in teenagers, it can briefly lead to mental instability due to a sudden offset or onset in hormone production.

It may also cause someone to lose confidence. In other words, it may cause the environment or conditions around the affected person to appear weak. The fact that the person is extremely vulnerable to several communicable diseases is another significant side effect. This happens because the loss of a crucial mineral for the body's defense mechanisms severely impairs the immune system. However, this can be avoided by taking zinc supplements or consuming foods high in zinc. Sore throats, rashes, skin infections, and various respiratory issues are a few of the infections that are frequently contracted.

The thyroid hormone occasionally fails to block the bones at the proper time, allowing them to grow more quickly. This frequently leads to tall people having thyroid issues that go untreated for a long time.

Chapter Six

How Sports Can Help to Improve a Girl's Self-Esteem

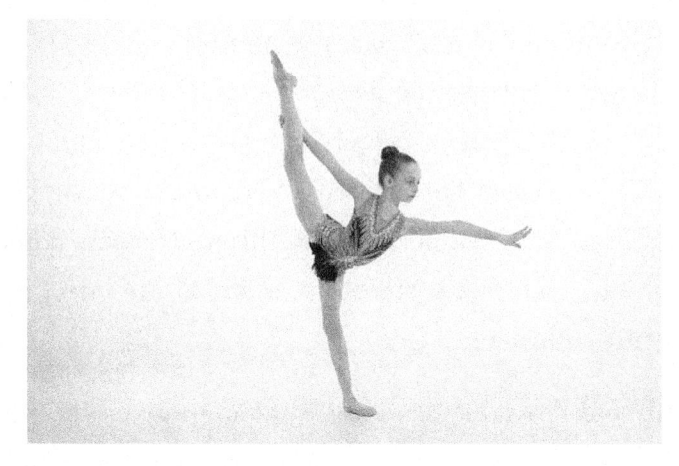

Playing sports was one of the few times my kids got to interact with other kids their age because I homeschooled them. I was willing to try any sport they wanted to because I enjoyed playing almost all sports. My daughter, who is now an adult and a bride, started playing softball when she was six years old. She realized she wasn't quite like most of the other girls over the course of the following couple of years. She appeared to be a still-baby-fatted, stunning young girl with rosy cheeks and blue eyes. She believed herself to be either overweight, slow, or clumsy. She was teased by some girls while being avoided by others. I observed that she wasn't by herself. Every team seemed to have at least a few players who didn't quite fit the stereotype.

I decided to restart my coaching career when she turned nine and started leading her softball teams so that she and every other girl would have a chance. I noticed that the majority of the coaches I saw were also parents of young girls who didn't quite fit the stereotype as I peered around at the other coaches. As a result, we were the coaches who were most familiar with the feelings of an outcast child. I identified my girl's strengths and assisted her in developing them so that she could fit in. Because of her incredibly strong arm, she mastered the positions of third base and catcher and developed into a respectable pitcher. She gained confidence as her teammates clapped for her rather than laughed at her, and she became more aware of her strengths.

These same girls, who were once made fun of, eventually developed into women who identified their specialties and put a lot of effort into honing them. They were the unpopular ones off the field. They were important links in the chain that made up their teams on the field, contributing to something greater than just outward appearances. These girls all discovered they had something to offer even during the challenging puberty years, and it was because of this that they felt bigger, better, and larger than life when they performed well on the field. No matter how they looked or where they came from, playing sports made them part of the "in" crowd. They were proud to be a part of the team, and this pride fueled their confidence, enabling them to accomplish more than they had anticipated!

We had a team near the end of my daughter's softball career that was roughly split into "popular" girls and "not-so-popular" girls. On the field, however, we were all together, and they realized that their teammates, coaches, and umpires all saw them as equals. They were all "somebody" out there. I had a core group of girls who had played ball together since they were young. For some of them, the field was the only place where they truly felt at home. My team of girls faced a formidable foe in the final game of the season, the championship game. Our team's "star" pitcher wasn't there that night, and our opponent's "star" pitcher (who also happened to be well-liked, well-known, and excellent at her position since she played varsity softball) had the potential to intimidate our players. However, our players didn't let that happen. They had learned that every girl had something unique to offer on the field and was proud to be a member of our unit when they stepped onto that diamond. We triumphed in that championship game against all odds because of the self-assurance these girls gained from playing softball over the years. My chunky friend left the room with assurance and threw a shutout. We scored the lone run in that game's 1-0 victory. One of those other underdog girls who just so happened to become a fast runner scored it. She was hit by a pitch, managed to steal second and third bases, and then scored from home on a wild pitch. The ones who left the field that night as big winners were two girls who played ball and built strong self-esteem!

They all discovered their strengths, received mentoring from encouraging coaches, and felt a part of something greater than themselves because these girls grew up playing sports together. They gained the self-assurance to carry themselves proudly. All girls can feel good about themselves while working together on a team, with the support of other girls who might not have considered them friends off the field. Girls who participate in sports learn that they can do and be anything they set their minds to, not just in the game of softball but in life as well.

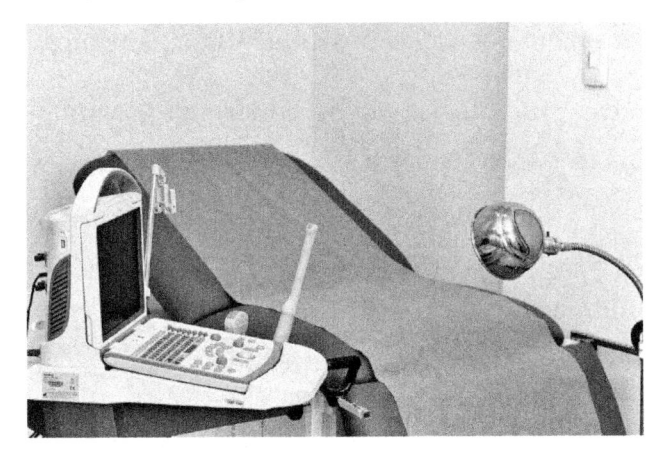

The Value of Taking a Young Girl to a Gynecologist

A young girl on the cusp of puberty should see a gynecologist in particular. These specialized medical professionals have received training specifically in female reproductive system care and potential issues. Teenage girls are likely to experience complex issues during this time, which calls for the assistance of a professional with expertise in that area. The majority of experts recommend that a young girl visit one of these specialists for the first time no later than a year after experiencing her first period. Although it can occur at any age between 9 and 15, it typically occurs around the age of 12. Even earlier or later periods occur for some girls.

A parent might want to make an appointment with a pediatric gynecologist, though it's not necessary. As they have experience treating adolescents, these doctors will be more receptive to inquiries and responses regarding the particular issues facing a young girl. Additionally, given that young girl is likely to be somewhat hesitant and afraid during their initial appointments, their bedside manner may be better suited to helping her.

A pediatric gynecologist will be better able to communicate these concerns to the patient and her parents because they have a keen understanding of what to expect from the developing and changing anatomy of an adolescent female. Naturally, a doctor who cares for both children and adults will have this expertise as well, though they might not be as adept at sharing their findings in this specific circumstance.

A young patient's opportunity to ask questions about their health and their reproductive system is provided by a visit to the gynecologist, in addition to helping to ensure that everything is functioning normally and there are no issues. A young girl might find it challenging to feel comfortable discussing these issues with her parents. A doctor will also be able to respond to inquiries about puberty and sexual development.

A good gynecologist who has experience treating young girls will also be able to respond to a wide range of queries about the health of teenagers. Once a young girl reaches this age, she is unlikely to visit the doctor regularly. If so, the girl may have the ideal opportunity to bring up issues specific to adolescence, like concerns about acne, drug use, smoking, and weight loss.

Chapter Seven

Discussing a Girl's First Period

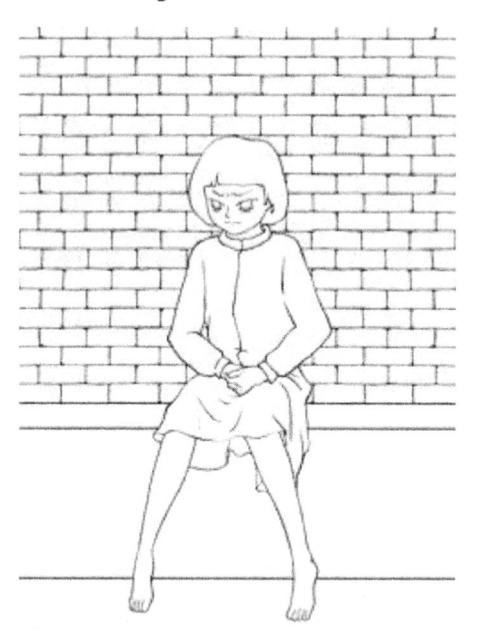

When should I start discussing my daughter's first period with her? How much information about the development, growth, and birth of a new sibling should I give my preschooler? Why does my eight-year-old son believe he is so knowledgeable about "the birds and the bees"? The family-friendly television program was full of suggestive sexual content. Should I have pushed for the switch to be turned off? How closely should I watch what my kids watch in the future?

These are just a few of the typical worries that parents have as their kids interact with a society that constantly sends them sexual messages. It is critical to understand the broader aspects of sexuality and the roles that family, friends, school, and the media play in influencing children's views of themselves as sexual beings to navigate the potential minefields between childhood and adult sexual identity safely and smoothly. Many parents wait until their child reaches puberty before talking about sexual issues. Some parents are forced to give their children "the talk" because of obvious physical changes in their children. Some parents are relieved when their child comes home clutching pamphlets distributed during a lecture on sex education because they are hoping the school will do what they don't want it to.

In addition, the majority of parents lack a strong background in the study of human sexuality. They might have hazy memories of their parents' awkward speeches, a book about a girl's first period, a book about human sexuality hidden in the back of the bookcase, or the week in health class that was devoted to reproduction. Given these conditions, it makes sense that parents frequently put off educating their children. Many parents also think their kids won't be interested in or tempted if they don't talk about it. But it is foolish to put off talking about sexuality until puberty or, worse yet, until your daughter has her first period. A child's sexuality is crucial to his or her development from the moment of birth and continues to be so throughout the rest of their life. The essence of parenting is providing children with the knowledge they need to make informed decisions and design their own life.

The same communication abilities that support healthy relationships between parents and children, in general, are needed when discussing sexuality. If parents can foster open discussions with their young children as they investigate sexuality together, this same openness will enable parents to provide advice and guidance as their children approach adolescence. The subject of sexuality will feel less natural for both parents and their children if they don't start the process early, and both may feel uncomfortable with this new intimacy and with the scope of the problems that need to be resolved quickly. But remember that starting late is much preferable to not starting at all.

I have also struggled with communication "how-tos," with the various interpretations of "the birds and the bees," and with the various facets of sexuality as a pediatrician and mother of three kids. The task has been challenging. I casually asked about the health curriculum before my oldest daughter started taking health classes at school. Her response alarmed me. I thought the curriculum, which would be taught by the male gym teacher, was insufficient. He was a nice guy, but I worried about my daughter, so I sheepishly offered my services. My offer to teach the class was quickly accepted, and as the relieved male teacher showered me with thanks and handed me the sparse curriculum, I suddenly felt anxious. As I got ready to lead the incredibly crucial class on puberty, menstruation, and conception, I had to overcome many obstacles. Changing my perspective on sexuality presented me with perhaps my biggest challenge. The subject is much more extensive than meets the eye. In addition to the mechanics of human reproduction, sexuality also encompasses relationships, morals, and a variety of life skills.

I was surprised by the students' resistance to turning to their families for support as I was teaching the health class. Even though they frequently said things like, "I am too embarrassed to speak to my mom about having my first period," these young girls were willing to ask a stranger for assistance. There was a chasm between mothers and daughters and parents and their kids. I felt there was a need to involve the entire family in the educational process. In response to this urge, I started a community class for mothers and their daughters. In it, we discussed the typical emotional and physical changes that occur during puberty as they both got ready for the girl's first period and all the ups and downs that come with it.

I found that mothers eagerly shared their worries with other mothers about the emotional turmoil they experienced with their maturing daughters and were excited to review the fundamental physiology of their daughters' physical changes. Similar to how the girls in the class had the chance to participate with their mothers, they were able to connect and build communication during an engaging educational process. This class served as a starting point for some families. There is undoubtedly a window of opportunity during these prepubertal years to open the door of communication about sexuality and to share your values with your children, even though it is best not to wait until puberty to bring up topics like a girl's first period. Think of classes where fathers and sons could interact similarly. Alternatively, why not have both parents attend the class with their kids?

What is the Right Age to Start Talking to Your Girl about Menstruation?

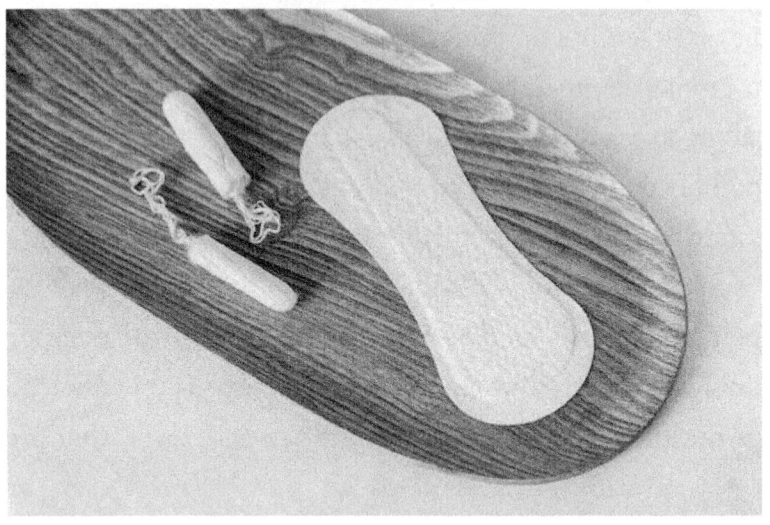

When should I start discussing my daughter's first period with her? How much information about a new sibling's development, growth, and birth should I give my preschooler? Why does my eight-year-old son believe he is so knowledgeable about "the birds and the bees"? The family-friendly television program was full of suggestive sexual content. Should I have pushed for the switch to be turned off? How closely should I watch what my kids watch in the future?

These are just a few of the typical worries that parents have as their kids interact with a society that constantly sends them sexual messages. It is critical to understand the broader aspects of sexuality and the roles that family, friends, school, and the media play in influencing children's views of themselves as sexual beings to navigate the potential minefields between childhood and adult sexual identity safely and smoothly. May parents wait until their child reaches puberty before talking about sexual issues. Some parents are forced to give their children "the talk" because of noticeable physical changes in their children. Some parents are relieved when their child comes home clutching pamphlets distributed during a lecture on sex education because they are hoping the school will do what they don't want it to.

In addition, the majority of parents lack a strong background in the study of human sexuality. They might have hazy memories of their parents' awkward speeches, a book about a girl's first period, a book about human sexuality hidden in the back of the bookcase, or the week in health class devoted to reproduction. Given these conditions, it makes sense that parents frequently put off educating their children. Many parents also think their kids won't be interested in sex or tempted if they don't talk about it. But it is foolish to put off talking about sexuality until puberty or, worse yet, until your daughter has her first period. A child's sexuality is crucial to his or her development from birth and continues to be so throughout the rest of their life. The essence of parenting is providing children with the knowledge they need to make informed decisions and design their own lives.

The same communication abilities that support healthy relationships between parents and children, in general, are needed when discussing sexuality. If parents can foster open discussions with their young children as they investigate sexuality together, this same openness will enable parents to provide advice and guidance as their children approach adolescence. The subject of sexuality will feel less natural for both parents and their children if they don't start the process early, and both may feel uncomfortable with this new intimacy and with the scope of the problems that need to be resolved quickly. But remember that starting late is much preferable to not starting at all.

I have also struggled with communication "how-to s," with the various interpretations of "the birds and the bees," and with the multiple facets of sexuality as a pediatrician and mother of three kids. The task has been challenging. I casually asked about the health curriculum before my oldest daughter started taking health classes at school. Her response alarmed me. I thought the curriculum, which the male gym teacher would teach, was insufficient. He was a nice guy, but I worried about my daughter, so I sheepishly offered my services. My offer to teach the class was quickly accepted, and as the relieved male teacher showered me with thanks and handed me the sparse curriculum, I suddenly felt anxious. As I got ready to lead the incredibly crucial class on puberty, menstruation, and conception, I had to overcome many obstacles. Changing my perspective on sexuality presented me with perhaps my biggest challenge. The subject is much more extensive than meets the eye.

In addition to the mechanics of human reproduction, sexuality also encompasses relationships, morals, and a variety of life skills.

I was surprised by the students' resistance to turning to their families for support as I was teaching the health class. Even though they frequently said things like, "I am too embarrassed to speak to my mom about having my first period," these young girls were willing to ask a stranger for assistance. There was a chasm between mothers and daughters and parents and their kids. I felt there was a need to involve the entire family in the educational process. In response to this urge, I started a community class for mothers and their daughters. In it, we discussed the typical emotional and physical changes that occur during puberty as they both got ready for the girl's first period and all the ups and downs that come with it.

I found that mothers eagerly shared their worries with other mothers about the emotional turmoil they experienced with their maturing daughters and were excited to review the fundamental physiology of their daughters' physical changes. Similar to how the girls in the class had the chance to participate with their mothers, they were able to connect and build communication during an engaging educational process. This class served as a starting point for some families. There is undoubtedly a window of opportunity during these prepubertal years to open the door of communication about sexuality and to share your values with your children, even though it is best not to wait until puberty to bring up topics like a girl's first period. Think of classes where fathers and sons could interact similarly. Alternatively, why not have both parents attend the class with their kids?

How to Predict the Arrival of Your Daughter's First Period

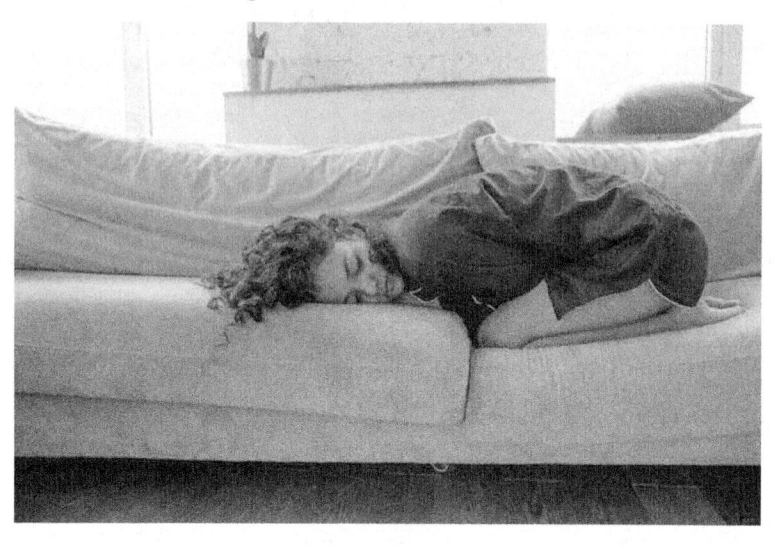

When our kids take their first steps, use their last diaper, or start school, it sometimes seems like as parents we are waiting and wondering when they will reach the next developmental milestone.

It's the same when your daughter goes through puberty. She will go through a lot of changes, including her menarche, or first period. Although no two children are alike and no one can predict with certainty when she will start getting her period, there are predictable stages of puberty that you can keep an eye on so that the two of you are both ready.

Even though internal changes can begin as early as age 8, the development of breast buds in girls marks the beginning of puberty around the ages of 11 to 12. When the nipples are just starting to rise, there are breast buds. In addition to developing in height and weight, girls of this age will also start to develop pubic hair, which initially appears fine and straight rather than curly.

For one to two years, the breast will continue to grow. Until her breasts are fully developed, they might feel tender and not be an even size. At this point, your daughter will start to experience vaginal discharge. You can reassure her that this is completely normal and that this is just how her body naturally cleanses itself. Remind yourself to consult your doctor if the discharge is dark in color or smells strong, as these characteristics may indicate an infection.

You can anticipate your daughter's period to start about two years after she first develops breast buds and has reached a weight of about 100 pounds. She may or may not exhibit any additional physical symptoms before her period; everyone differs. She will most likely only become aware that she has begun menstruating during a routine trip to the restroom. But the more she is aware of puberty and the physical changes it brings about, the less shocked she will be on the big day.

Your daughter may experience specific symptoms once her period begins. Although almost all girls have periods, not all girls have the same experience. While some girls can easily get through their monthly periods pain-free, others deal with a variety of physical issues that make menstruation uncomfortable.

Premenstrual syndrome is the most typical symptom experienced during the monthly cycle (PMS). A week or so before the start of menstruation, a group of symptoms known as PMS may have some bearing on your life. PMS symptoms frequently include:

- Bleeding in the abdomen
- Breast tenderness or smelliness
- Stress or anxiety
- Trouble sleeping
- Joint or muscle pain
- Headache
- Fatigue
- Acne or worsening of pre-existing skin conditions
- Changes in mood

Despite the widespread belief that most women have some PMS symptoms, very few women have these symptoms.

Another period symptom is cramping. The endometrium, the mucous membrane that lines the uterus, is shed during menstruation as a result of the uterus contracting or tightening. Some girls may find this to be unsettling or even painful.

Consult your family doctor for suggestions on improving things better if your daughter's daily activities are being hampered by PMS symptoms or cramps.

Your daughter might also have irregular menstrual cycles. The average girl will need at least a year to get used to a "regular" 28-day cycle, though this can range from 21 to 45 days. Menstruation can range from light to heavy during the first year, lasting a few days one month and longer the next. It is also common to miss one or two months.

With a calendar and notes on the type of flow experienced, you can assist your daughter in keeping track of her periods. If you are worried about your daughter's pattern, speak to your family doctor.

Your daughter will feel empowered to take care of her health and have control over her monthly experience if you can help her understand and manage any period-related symptoms she may experience.

Getting Your Girl Ready for Her Period

It is crucial to treat a young girl's first experience with her period, or menstruation, as it is more commonly known, as a milestone.

Too frequently, mothers treat their daughters as though they are at fault for going through it. Yes, too many mothers assume that their young daughters understand what "having their period" means. She wasn't even informed enough to anticipate it. Yes, she was not informed of anything. And to top it all off, the child is made to feel "senseless" for not being aware of it.

Due to her fear and confusion on that particular day, the young girl begins to resent this significant aspect of her femininity.

This attitude needs to change, and it can if every mother makes the effort to get her daughter ready for this unique occasion. This article should be useful in this regard.

The Proper Moment

Usually, a young girl's first period begins between the ages of twelve and fourteen. However, it can happen to anyone at any age even as young as eight or as old as sixteen.

Therefore, as she grows, be aware of all the minor and significant changes that her body will experience. Since we do not yet know the precise day that it will occur, this will allow you to roughly estimate when it will occur. Her emotional state must also be taken into account. In other words, is she prepared for this discussion? Let's move on to the following suggestion after taking these two factors into account:

Pose and Respond To Inquiries

You can start by asking her if she is aware of what it is, and if she is, then you can ask her to share with you what she is aware of. The response may astound you.

Correct any misunderstandings without passing judgment.

Describe its cause and expected duration. Define a pad and a tampon, and describe how she can and must maintain her hygiene during this time.

Do not forget that she may experience cramps, headaches, constipation, diarrhea, and other symptoms throughout her entire body.

A Visual Aid

Show her how to properly wear a pad and some underwear. Show her where you keep yours and encourage her to carry a few pads with her on walks in case she needs them if she is away from home.

Give her a chance to practice; make sure she wears it while walking around; and offer her as many pointers as you can. For instance, she should wear two pairs of underwear and dark clothing instead of white during these times if she feels uncomfortable wearing just one.

Save Some Cramps For Later

You do not need to cover everything in this one conversation, though. As the days pass, space it out, and be sure to state clearly that you want to know how she is doing from month to month.

You should take her to the doctor if she is experiencing more cramps than usual. Mothers sometimes disregard their daughters' stomachaches because they believe they are common. Take her to the doctor if the cramps are too much for her.

Together, Spend Time

On the first day, you and she can stay in and relax at home while watching TV, reading, or just eating and chatting until she nods off.

There is nothing for her to be afraid of, so take as much of the fear out of it as you can for her.

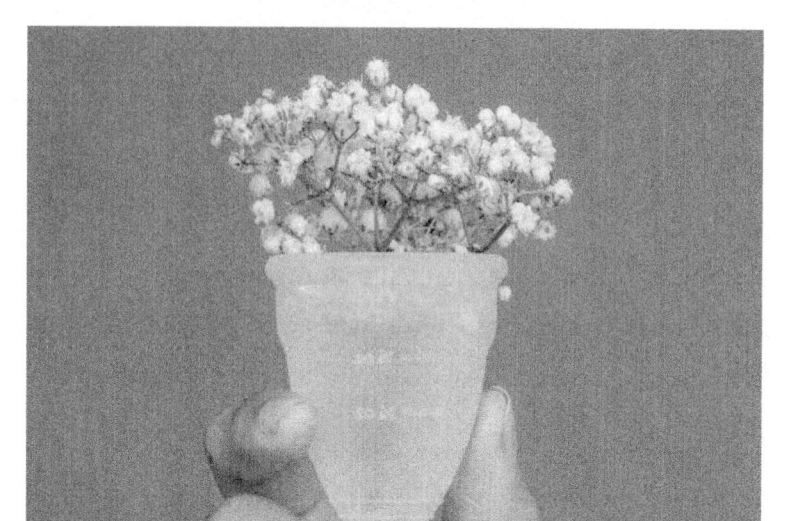

Her First Period

Your adorable little girl is maturing and becoming a woman. You want to get her ready for the day she gets her first period because you can see the warning signs.

You don't feel entirely at ease about it, and you're unsure of how to start or what to say. This is entirely understandable given that discussing menstruation is taboo and has always been so.

Most parents find it challenging to have frank conversations with their daughters about the changes that come with puberty because of this.

To help you approach this time with confidence, I have put together a few suggestions.

1. Know Your Material First.

A good way to overcome the taboo is to be well-informed and aware of exactly what happens during menstruation. The more familiar you are with your "material," the more at ease you will be speaking about it. You have access to a wealth of printed and online resources.

Your daughter will need to comprehend the following from a purely physical or biological standpoint:

- The mechanisms of female bleeders
- What happens to their changing body every month
- What women use (types, brands, alternatives), and how they use it to catch the flow
- Simple pain relief
- How to record and monitor a cycle
- Fertility fundamentals

Be selective about what your daughter needs to know at any stage because girls are starting their periods at a younger age. Young girls (10 or 11 years old) require simpler information than older girls (14 or 15 years old).

Opening up lines of communication and making information accessible will help them take in what they can.

Helping your younger daughter deal with the physical aspects might be a top priority if you have one. For instance, how to use it, the timing of periods, etc.

At this point, she doesn't need to be aware of her fertility, but you can certainly lay the groundwork for a later conversation. You can inform her that her body sends signals to let her know when it is fertile, that each stage of the cycle serves a specific function, and that as she gets older, she will be able to learn to recognize the unique signals her body is sending her.

Menstruation should be considered from both a physical and an emotional standpoint, in addition to the former. After all, your daughter's next big challenge, and one that also affects those around her will be learning to manage her emotions and her physicality after she has the facts and her physicality under control.

2. Remove Your Sensitivity.

Take it from me: the more you discuss and consider menstruation, the more commonplace it seems. For the past ten years, I have written about and talked about menstruation; to me, it is just a natural part of life. So exercise. Before trying it on your daughter, practice on your spouse or close friends. In doing so, you'll feel less embarrassed, which will immediately ensure a much better outcome.

3. The Value of Self-Awareness.

Being conscious of your own emotions and ideas regarding menstruation is crucial. Everybody has ingrained beliefs, often negative ones, about what menstruation signifies. A portion of the discomfort and embarrassment you may experience can be alleviated by taking the time to consider and reframe your attitude toward menstruation.

Now is the time to reconsider the menstrual cycle if you are a woman and your transition into puberty was marked by shame and rejection. Do you want your daughter to continue this unfortunate family tradition? What do your daughter's development and sexual maturation mean to you?

If your daughter is in the early stages of puberty, it may be particularly challenging to answer the second question. The abundance of synthetic hormones in our diets and a more sedentary lifestyle are contributing to girls starting their periods at younger and younger ages.

It's crucial to keep in mind that just because your daughter's body is developing, it doesn't necessarily follow that her mind or emotions will follow suit. There is time to adjust because the entire puberty process can last a couple of years. And just because your daughter has her period doesn't mean that she will automatically start acting sexually.

What do you feel?

Childhood fades into the past as adolescents enter a new stage of development. Many emotions surfaced during times of change or transition, as there always are. Grief over time lost, fear for the future, rage at outside forces, or our aging process as our daughters enter their prime are all valid emotions.

It's not a simple time. You are less likely to become embroiled in conflicts and are better able to tenderly support your daughter through her transition if you are open to your own conflicting emotions and can put them in perspective.

4. Continue To Communicate Effectively.

When they need to talk, be ready to do so. It's amusing when we get all pumped up to have this really important conversation with our children only to find out they're not interested at all. Then, unexpectedly, at a later date, they are prepared and catch us off, guard.

When the chance to speak arises, seize it. Be prepared with your knowledge and remember that they frequently require information in small, manageable chunks. If you can't tell them the entire story at once, try not to get too upset.

Another effective tactic is to keep books easily accessible throughout the home so that your child can get the information for themselves Remember that resources are available for you as well when using these books as the basis for discussions.

Chapter Eight

Breast and Bra

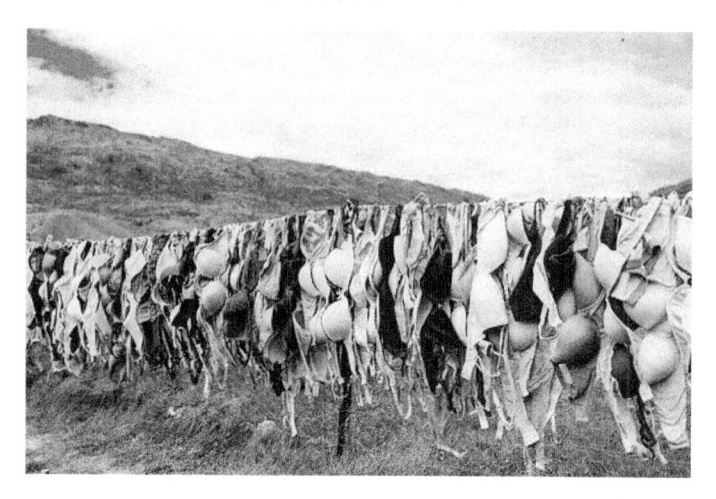

Your Daughter's Health & Breast Growth

Every young girl experiences excitement when she first becomes aware of her body's changes and the beginnings of her breast development. Breasts are designed to produce milk for nursing infants, but in today's society, they are also viewed as a sign of readiness for sexual activity.

Have no fear if your teenage daughter starts to inquire about her breasts; a young girl's curiosity about her breasts is completely normal. She will probably have questions about what might go wrong, how big she can anticipate them getting, and how they will look. Here are a few straightforward responses that you can give to any teenage girl who starts posing queries:

Both a woman's diet and any genes she may have can affect how her breasts develop.

Within two arduous stages of a woman's life, puberty and when she becomes pregnant, she can anticipate that her breasts will expand to a discernible size.

Once she first starts puberty, a woman's body begins to mature. Her breasts should begin developing at this point in terms of size and shape. While some girls may not notice any change until they are around 13 or 14, other girls may not notice any change until they are around 7 years old. Of course, each girl is unique, and it just depends on your internal biological "clock."

Once her internal signals are received, she will start to notice a change. The first sign inside is when her pituitary gland instructs her body to begin producing estrogen. The fat that is deposited in the breast from the production of estrogen is what causes the breast to begin growing. After that, the woman's milk ducts will expand, which will cause the breasts to grow even bigger.

Always keep in mind that a woman's nutrition, health, and hormone levels all have an impact on the size of her breasts. She can get a good idea of when she should expect to experience puberty by looking at her family history and the date of her mother's first period. Teenage girls will notice that their breasts are shrinking if they follow a very poor diet and lose a lot of weight.

Her breasts will start to grow again once she starts eating better and getting healthier. Remember that even after she turns 18, her breasts won't be fully developed until she goes through pregnancy. Her breasts will continue to grow and develop until then.

The size of her breasts is ultimately influenced by her genetics and heredity.

Her breasts can be anywhere between a small bra size (like an AA) and a large bra size (like a DD). Of course, everything depends on her genetics, diet, and potential body type. Keep in mind that each breast's growth will not always be the same. She might have one breast that is bigger than the other until her breasts are fully developed, but don't worry, her smaller breast will catch up!

The milk ducts inside her breasts will begin to produce milk once she has gone through a pregnancy. This will get her ready to breastfeed her new child. Keep in mind that breast growth is significant; it is not just a matter of society or vanity. She needs her breasts for a variety of reasons, and now that she understands why and how to care for them, she's more likely to live a longer life free of illness! Always conduct breast self-examinations to look for lumps or other breast cancer warning signs on your daughter. With liquid vitamins, you can boost your health while giving her more energy.

What Your Young Girl Should Know About Bra Types

Oh, the bra. This once-basic article of clothing has evolved into a symbol of femininity. The science of the bra has advanced tremendously, giving us incredible support and unmatched comfort in a variety of styles, sizes, fabrics, and shapes.

We'll talk about the different kinds of bras available. They can be flashy or practical, sexy or supportive, or novelty- or nursing-oriented. You're probably familiar with some of them. Other people might all be strangers to you. So join us as we explore the fantastic world of the brasserie. You might even come out with a little more business knowledge than you had before.

"The Classics"

A training bra is made for young girls whose breasts are just starting to develop. It is significantly smaller than typical cup sizes and typically does not include underwire support. While girls adjust to wearing a bra, it merely offers a minimal amount of support.

The full-cup bra is a useful daily bra that covers the majority of the breasts. This bra offers a lot of support and comfort, making it especially suitable for women with larger breasts.

A half-cup style, the demi-cup bra extends just past the nipples. It goes well with shirts or dresses that have deeper necklines and can be worn by women with breasts of all sizes.

A wire wraps around the breast's lower half in an *underwired bra*. Although the wire supports the wearer and aids in maintaining the bra's shape, some women find underwire bras uncomfortable.

Instead of using an underwire, the soft-cup bra uses a sturdy band to provide support. *A soft-cup bra* is more comfortable for many women.

The strapless bra pairs well with shirts and dresses that show shoulders because it lacks shoulder straps.

The back shoulder straps of *the racerback bra* are arranged in a V pattern. The straps fit better under some shirts and dresses because they are close to the neck.

Those who "function"

Women who engage in *physical activity* in particular are the target market for the sports bra. They fit snugly and hold the breasts in place, so they are supportive and comfortable even during the most strenuous exercise.

The *maternity bra* can be adjusted to accommodate a woman's changing breast size and weight during pregnancy. It enlarges to allow for breast sensitivity and development.

To make breastfeeding simpler, the *nursing bra* was developed. Nursing bras are designed with easily removable flaps, unlike conventional bras, which aren't exactly feeding-friendly.

For women who had one or both breasts removed due to cancer, the *mastectomy bra* was created. To give the appearance of natural breasts, the bra has special cups that can hold breast prostheses.

Those who "enhance"

The padded bra resembles a standard bra but has some additional padding in the cup linings. This gives the impression that the breasts are slightly bigger or fuller.

The push-up bra is made to enhance the cleavage the most. It has a distinctive design with a lot of padding intended to lift and bind the breasts. The padding may occasionally be a part of the lining; alternatively, silicone or water inserts may be used.

Women with very large busts, typically over 34C, should use *the minimizer bra*. The minimizer bra shapes and compresses the breasts to give them a smaller appearance while also increasing comfort and support.

To fit into a wedding gown, *the bridal bra* is a corset that shapes the waist. This type of bra supports the breasts comfortably and encourages good posture.

The "Novelties"

The shelf bra hardly covers any breasts at all; it is merely a band that runs beneath them. This bra is more of a sexual accessory than one that offers any support.

Additionally, *a peephole bra* is used in intimate situations. The peephole bra has holes that allow the nipples to be seen, but it does cover most of the breasts.

The third type of erotic bra is *the cupless bra*. It is a brassiere frame without cups, allowing the nipples to be prominently displayed.

The last type of bra that is more for show than for function is *the novelty bra*. Novelty bras are made of unusual materials like shells or coconuts and are frequently worn as accessories with costumes.

'New Fangled'

The straps on *the convertible bra* can be removed and rearranged to match the style or cut of your clothing, making it a useful bra to keep in your wardrobe. Transparent straps are also offered on some convertible bras.

The built-in bra is sewn into a shirt or dress's framework. They offer some support, usually in the form of an elastic band, but on occasion, a full underwire frame is used.

The t-shirt bra is intended to be undetectable. Because there are no raised seams, the garment sits smoothly without exposing bra lines when a woman wears a tight shirt.

The cleverly designed *u-plunge bra* offers exceptional support even when wearing a deep plunging neckline. Even with extremely low necklines, the u-plunge style is invisible because it connects low on the chest.

Since *the adhesive bra* has no straps or bands, it doesn't offer support. It's designed to go with clothing that has no back. Some adhesive bras are paper-based and are only meant to be used once.

Others are washable and reusable because they are made of silicone. Both attach to the breasts using a powerful adhesive.

Choosing the correct bra

Choosing the ideal bra for yourself and your girl can be challenging. It's important to have both a variety of properly fitting bras and occasion-appropriate bras on hand. Sports bras that offer enough support for your various activities are essential if you are a regular jogger or athlete. If an expectant mother intends to breastfeed, she should buy a selection of nursing bras.

Every few years, it's a good idea to get your bra fitted because breasts change over time. You can get a more precise fit than trying to measure yourself at one of the many lingerie stores that offer assistance with bra sizing. You might be shocked to learn that you've been wearing the wrong size bra for years if you've never had one fitted.

While wearing clothing that doesn't fit properly can be uncomfortable, it can also lead to more serious issues like backaches. So before purchasing any new bras, it's a good idea to get an accurate bra size.

Examining Young Girls' Risk for Breast Cancer and Self-Protection Strategies

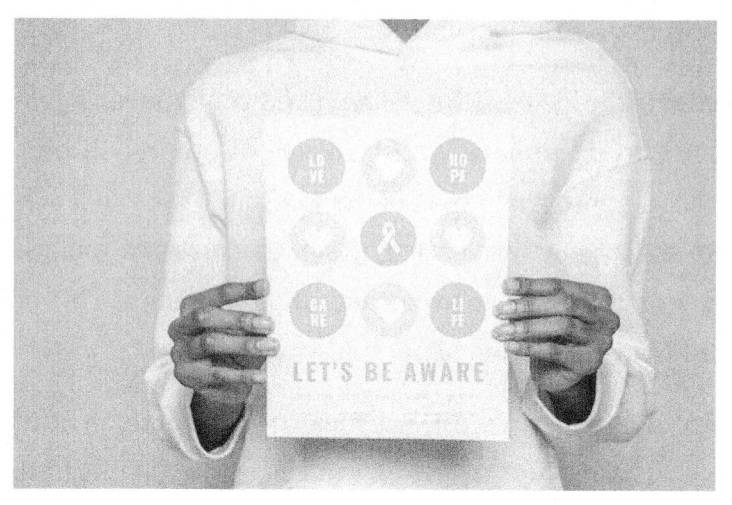

Most likely, a lot of people are curious if breast cancer can affect young girls. It is true that it can, even though it is uncommon during puberty. One in every 231 women under the age of 40 is at risk for developing breast cancer, but most of those women are at least thirty years old. However, breast lumps in young adults are typical. This blatant contradiction can be explained by the fact that teenagers frequently develop benign breast tumors or cysts in response to estrogen sensitivity. These lumps frequently go away on their own, but it is often a good idea to have them checked out by a doctor.

Doctors frequently recommend waiting for three menstrual cycles after finding a lump before taking any further action because the likelihood is high that it will go away.

In adolescents, mammograms or breast x-rays are typically not required.

Gynecologists frequently teach breast self-examination techniques to teenagers, so by the time they are in their forties and at a higher risk of breast cancer, this can become a healthy habit. Birth control pill use has been shown to lower the risk of developing benign breast tumors, indicating that it won't make it more likely for adolescents to develop breast cancer.

Although it is unlikely for young people to get breast cancer, it is still a good idea to learn about your breasts and how to spot any problems.

Learning about breast cancer early on can undoubtedly make a significant difference if you ever develop it.

You should have a breast exam performed by a medical professional once every year or two once your breasts start to develop. Though opinions on how frequently to get one vary among experts, you should probably get one at least once a year. Allowing a doctor to examine your breasts can also be a little embarrassing, but keep in mind that the doctor doesn't think much of it. It's very helpful and only takes a minute or two, and it might just save your life.

Make sure to check your breasts once a month to look for any changes or indications of breast cancer or other issues. A breast self-exam, or BSE for short, is what this is. Since it's common for breasts to become slightly swollen and uncomfortable before or during a menstrual period, try to do it as soon as possible after you've had your period. A BSE will help women find cysts or other benign breast issues in between exams. This may help some women recognize breast cancer, which is uncommon in young adults in particular. A BSE can be completed quickly and easily; it usually only takes a few minutes. BSE is a technique you can use for the rest of your life to help ensure you have excellent breast health, although it seems strange or inopportune.

Young adults should be aware of several signs and symptoms of breast cancer, such as ridges or thickened patches of skin on the breast or nipple area, inversion of the nipple, breast soreness, a change in breast size or appearance, a lump or swelling under the armpit, discharge from the nipple, dimpled skin on the breast, etc. Make a quick appointment with a general practitioner if you notice any of these red flags or any other unusual changes.

Chapter Nine

Choosing the Right Foods

10 Surprising Methods for Raising a Healthy Eater: Real Food, Real Kids, and Real Love

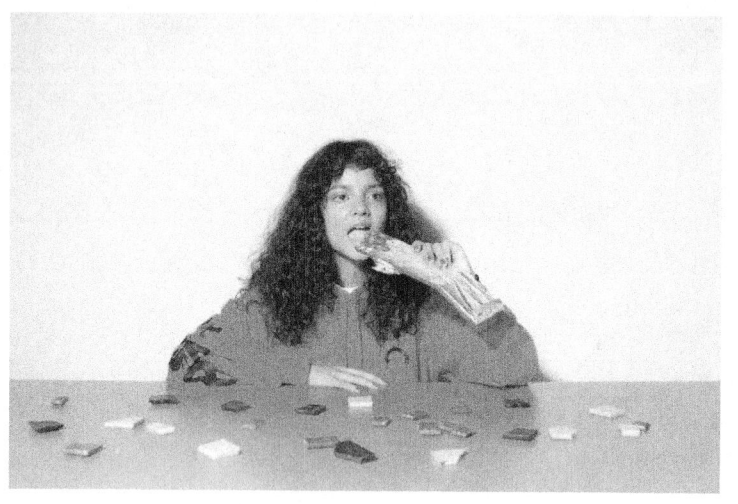

Almost nothing bothers us more than the food choices that our children make. The underlying parental fear is the same whether you're worried about raising a picky eater, a carb-junkie, or a veggie-phobe: that we can control our children's tastes if we have the right advice and food available. Then we spend our money on things like self-help books, cookware, kitchen utensils (slap chop, anyone?), and most importantly, our time, stress, and energy. We commit suicide in the kitchen, feel guilty about our "failures," and chastise our partners and family members for undermining our carefully planned efforts. Sounds recognizable?

The fact is that every child is unique. Their palates develop at various rates, just like how they grow and mature.

With that being said,

10 essential truths for raising children who eat healthfully for the rest of their lives

1. Real children require real food.

The farmer's market peach was enjoyed by my daughter. She also enjoys the farmer's market peach too.

Whether you are a vegan or an omnivore, sharing real food with your children is beneficial. Simple logic dictates that the closer the food is to the plant, the better it is. Raw ingredients always win over processed food. Don't buy something if someone is actively attempting to sell it to you on television or if it is made of shiny plastic and cartoon characters. Avoid putting ingredients in your mouth if you can't pronounce them. Red food dyes are prohibited in the EU because they can lead to ADHD-related behaviors, but they are present in almost everything in crinkly packaging here.

2. Real children don't have any extras.

Some parents find this concept to be problematic. Many of the mothers I know invest a lot of money in supplements and take pride in including anything their children eat in their diets, from spinach in spaghetti sauce to protein powder in smoothies. Although we adore adding a bunch of beets to a pot of chili, If this practice stresses you (or your wallet) out, it is not worth it. I'm not completely against it. I would be much more cautious when taking any supplements after the lead-tainted gummi bears vitamin scare, though, in the interest of full disclosure, my daughter enjoys fish oil "chewies" regularly. However, in the end, the emotional connection you make with food matters much more than the food's actual nutritional value. Do what you can within reason, then celebrate your success.

3. Real kids do experience "food binges."

My daughter has only wanted applesauce to eat for the past four weeks. The previous item was hummus. Avocadoes. Gummi Bears (I prefer not to discuss those times). Food tantrums are a common occurrence in childhood, especially after toddlerhood. Like a cherished blanket or bear, many psychologists think it's a child's way of creating consistency and security.

The only effective way to handle food rages is to wait them out while providing alternatives. I'm sure applesauce will be outmoded one day. The "it" food will be something else. Similar to how rockstars and starlets will be when she enters her oh-so-fun tween years.

According to nutritionists, it can take up to 20 exposures for a child to try a new food for the first time, without nagging, guilt, or pressure. I realize that's a tall order, but I've seen it work wonders during my daughter's crazily picky phases. I gave her avocado 12 times, and on the 12th time, it became her go-to meal for the first time in six weeks without nagging, guilt, or pressure. I realize that's a tall order, but I've seen it work wonders during my daughter's crazily picky phases. I gave her an avocado 12 times, and on the 12th time, it became her go-to meal for the next six weeks. In this home, avocado has reached platinum status!

4. Real children consume real milk.

Generally speaking, I don't recommend any specific foods or eating habits to my clients because I want them to do what is right for them and their families. I followed a low-meat diet for 14 years while putting great emphasis on both my health and vitality as well as the health of the planet. However, I firmly believe that there are a variety of healthy eating strategies and that you are on the right track as long as you feel good. Having said that, I don't often witness a food-based miracle like this one. When my daughter was 10 months old, she was diagnosed with asthma, she was wheezing almost constantly and was on a combination of breastmilk and formula (pump supply issues are a long story). After months of testing, she was put on a nebulizer with potent steroids and we were instructed to switch her to a "hypoallergenic" formula. I realized I couldn't do it after taking just one look at the materials. First on the list of ingredients was high-fructose corn syrup. Then a long, ominous list of broken-down protein chains, fats, and various unpronounceable chemicals appeared. UGH! This garbage was prescribed to us. I started doing some serious research while working extremely hard to increase my supply. As an experienced researcher, I knew I had made a significant discovery because what I discovered was astounding. The size is likely outside the purview of this book. I hesitantly joined my first co-op for raw milk and brought home my first gallon of unpasteurized whole milk. Because Organic Pastures wasn't yet widely available at Whole Foods, everything felt very cloak and dagger. I switched to only raw dairy products for my daughter and myself after she had just experienced a very wheezy first birthday. I entertained daily fantasies of ER visits and CPS officers knocking on my door because I wasn't sure if I was going to kill or cure us.

Then it took place. My dairy-daredevil experiment lasted less than a week before the wheezing stopped, and it has yet to return. When he listened to her lungs a month later, her allergist started crying. Since then, I haven't stopped yelling into the sky about how amazing raw, unprocessed milk from healthy, content cows is.

5. Actual children don't always eat their vegetables, they are watching to see if you do!

One of those things that ought to be obvious but need to be corrected is this. Okay, this will seem like a big tangent, but I assure you that it isn't:

Widespread of the campaign has encouraged parents to read aloud to their children for almost three decades. Reading aloud to kids is supposed to help them become better readers. However, a recent study demonstrates that it is entirely ineffective; kids who are read to for 30 minutes or more every day perform no better than their peers who are not read to. Yikes! How were those hours spent with Dora and Boots? Yes, folks, that's time I'll never get back.

So what triggers a child to start reading? The study discovered that a parent who read books themselves and frequently told their children, "Don't bother me, I'm reading," was the only factor that could create legions of lifelong bookworms. So start reading that book you've been meaning to! (Oh, and thanks to Mom for her beloved mysteries, which helped me become the academic force I am today.)

I'd argue that we both need to adopt a "Don't bother me, I'm eating!" mentality when it comes to food. So your child refuses to eat vegetables? Then what? Do you consume your own? with vigor? Kids will frequently act by our actions rather than our stated intentions. That irritates me.

6. Real kids, head back to the garden.

No, not the kind of stardust-golden hippie. The hands-in-the-dirt, fresh, sweet burst of flavor is a tomato variety that comes directly from the vine. Spending time cultivating vegetables is the most effective way to give your children an advantage in leading a life full of great vegetable goodness.

This was the focus of my research at Oxford. I could see that nutrition education was doomed to failure, even though billions of dollars had been spent on it in our public schools. Simply put, it is ineffective to advise children to avoid unhealthy foods and stick to nutritious ones. They might alter their routines for a day or two, maybe even a week, and then go back to eating Mountain Dew and red-hot Cheetos. That was the question I asked.

I then began delving deeply into marketing research. This is scary stuffy in marketing research. This is really scary stuff. The food marketing industry has known for 50 years that eating is all about how food makes you feel, not how food fuels your body, which nutritionists either overlook or ignore. And yes, that's essentially the focus of this entire website; adults can also benefit from it. But man, did these businesses know how to cheer us up? ("I adore it!")

What can be done to change that, then? Although it may seem overwhelming, there is one glimmer of hope among the mountains of research I've done on various nutrition education strategies for trying to stem the tide: farm and garden programs. These were unique programs. They got kids outside in the sun and dirt, which is where most kids want to be anyway, and helped them experience fresh, healthy food from a different angle, rather than trying to browbeat kids into healthy eating with fears of obesity and premature death. When you cultivate, tend to, prepare, and consume a vegetable, you develop a lifelong emotional bond with it. It would be best if you did not use your mind when eating. Blueberries were the first plant I ever successfully grew on my own, on a condo patio, at the tender age of 29, so I still have an almost unnatural enthusiasm for them.

I was inspired to start Full Circle Farm by this simple fact, and I've been fortunate to witness this amazing phenomenon firsthand. I brought a group of ten sixth graders to the farm, and they were harvesting their first patch of vegetables ever, a raggedy patch of somewhat overgrown radishes from the educational garden. They had never eaten a radish before (yes, you read that right). They all simultaneously took bites. These radishes were enormous, and anyone familiar with radishes is aware that large radishes have a woody, spicy flavor. Oh, my God, now that I've done it, I'm thinking as I'm on my knees next to the garden patch. They won't ever consume anything that we grow here again. Chewing was prevalent. Several wrinkled noses she then grinned. Smiles! I try one after deciding I must be mistaken. Blech! I had to control my urge to spit it out. The radishes were a favorite among all ten of my students; they all insisted remained eating them for the remainder of the time. I kept chuckling to myself the rest of the day. Red-hot Cheetos, take that. You're going down, Mountain Dew.

So make sure that you and your kids start a garden, whether it's a carrot growing in an old rainboot or a full-on homestead operation!

7. Real kids eat it at least a few times a week.

As you may have noticed, I did not say *every day, real life is damned* but let's be honest and admit that many of us lead busy lives that prevent us from always being on time and sitting down to dinner every night of the week. However, the majority of us are capable of doing better. A few weeks of family meals at the table can improve children's eating habits and strengthen family bonds in ways other activities cannot. The loudest sound at your dinner table is a cricket. That is undoubtedly a sign that you need to stay longer there, but don't worry, help is available! With verbal games and conversation starters, you can make it enjoyable.

Having to deal with a grumpy teen? Even more justification for eating three to four times per week. In a groundbreaking study, researchers showed that teens who ate at least three (not six or seven; busy mothers!) meals a week at a family dinner table had an incredibly different mentality toward food, including:

- Healthier eating (eating more vegetables and drinking less soda).
- Improved literacy (dinner conversation, anyone?)
- They have a risk of developing an eating disorder that is less than half that of peers without a family table.
- A decrease in risky behaviors
- Positive feelings about spending time with family, which they admitted to the research team but lied to their parents about.

Why not try ringing the dinner bell in a high-tech way?

8. Sincere kids get fat, then skinny, then fat, then skinny, etc.

Don't react inappropriately if your child starts to get a little chunky, please. Limiting sugar and junk food intake is always a good idea, but calling attention to your child's weight gain can humiliate and damage her already delicate body image (yeah, I'm talking to you).

What should we replace it with? Examine yourself in the mirror. No, not to remind yourself of how obscenely fat you've become! Reflect on how you were treated as a child and determine why you feel this way. Was that approach helpful for my self-image? Will treating my child in the same manner that I did (especially if it involves continuing a pattern of condescension and control) benefit her in any way?

You will need to be especially careful about how you respond to your child's very normal development over the years if you grew up in a home where gaining weight was considered shameful. Also, keep in mind that most girls gain a lot of weight right before puberty because their bodies work overtime to help them reach the 13% body fat requirement necessary to start their period's concerns. Fortunately for them, this is also the time of day when they are most sensitive to their weight and body type. So be cautious. Consider your child's heart before his body.

9. Real kids don't watch commercials.

So I'm assuming that by now you can tell that I think food marketers are terrible. The only way to humiliate them is to ensure that their $1.6 billion in advertising spending is wasted. A commercial-free childhood should be the goal of every health-conscious parent, even though some advertisements are so pervasive that it can be challenging to avoid them. Studies have shown that food advertisements on television are typically calorie- and nutrient-free junk food fests. Therefore, stop the commercials and possibly even the TV. Since giving up television two years ago, we haven't looked back, without TV or other media. This home has a lot of media consumption going on between iTunes, Netflix, and YouTube. We simply avoid advertisements. The tremendous side effect? In addition to not being sold, my life feels much less chaotic. It takes about a week of not watching network television for someone to realize how loud everyone is. What's going on there? In any case, a quick remote reflex and a TIVO will also work.

10. Children with real parents need them.

Have you ever caught your kid staring at you? Now, think back, parents of teenagers. Your child will look up at you with complete and utter adoration during the years before puberty when the hormone-induced "I hate you" fits that involve slamming doors and rolling eyes will occur. These heartbreakingly tender moments, the kiss on the cheek, the tender glance, the warm embrace, have all happened to us. Nothing is a better mirror for how you should feel about yourself than this. It is the foundation of the parent-child relationship. Your kid is aware that you are the most remarkable, attractive, courageous, and wonderful person on the planet. Why are you unable to concur with him? Maybe you can?

Rarely do people have constant feelings of self-worth. On the other hand, our children serve as a powerful, reciprocal mirror for us parents. We can mirror our child's unwavering love for us and progress toward self-acceptance by showing ourselves the same love. Everyone loves us, and everyone who loves us demonstrates it. We are flawless. Not in 10 years, not in 10 pounds, not when you fit into your skinny jeans.

A Teenage Girl's Guide to 50 Safe Pounds of Weight Loss

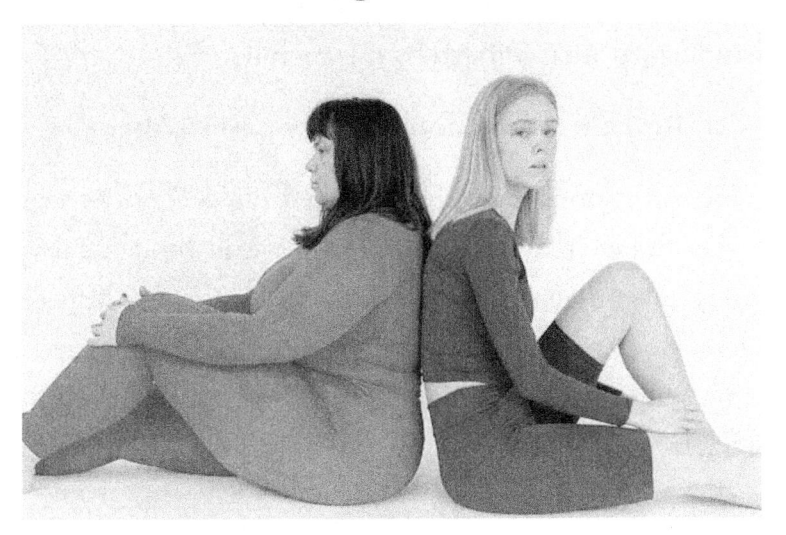

Every girl aspires to have a trim, slim body. However, weight gain begins before you enter your adolescent years. The main cause of a sudden increase in height and size is puberty. An increase in caloric intake, bingeing on junk and fast food, and a lack of exercise are additional causes of the issue.

Teenage weight gain is, in some ways, uncontrollable, but some lifestyle choices can be made to keep an eye on weight. Teenagers who want to lose weight must also be careful about the steps they take, as the body is still in a growth phase and cannot be denied proper nutrition. Here are some quick and safe ways to lose weight if you're a teen who wants to shed your chubby frame.

1. **Set a sensible objective.**

The majority of obese and overweight teenagers want to lose weight quickly, but it's important to take it slowly. For teenagers, 2 pounds per week is a reasonable amount. Long-term fat loss and weight maintenance are facilitated by this method.

2. Refrain from choosing low-calorie diets.

Reducing calories helps with weight loss. For teenagers, the quickest way to reduce their calorie intake is through fad and crash diets. Since they concentrate on one food category while excluding others, fat diets are not healthy choices. Once you resume your old eating patterns, the pounds start to creep back on. Rather than following fad diets, you can reduce your daily calorie intake by a specific percentage.

3. A wholesome diet.

During the teen years, an adolescent's body experiences significant developmental changes. Consequently, getting the right kind of nutrition is important. In addition to providing the body with the nutrients it needs, a balanced diet that contains the right amounts of fiber, lean protein, vitamins, and unsaturated fat also helps people stay at a healthy weight. Teenagers should eat fewer trans-fat, sugar, and sodium-rich foods and more fruits and vegetables. Eat as many freshly prepared meals and unprocessed, uncooked foods as you can.

4. Physical Exercise.

If teenagers maintain a healthy diet and exercise frequently, they can lose 50 pounds more quickly.

Although a teen's exercise program for weight loss should be customized to meet their unique physical needs and abilities and include cardiovascular and strength training exercises, it should be similar to that of an adult. Some cardiovascular exercises you should do include swimming, dancing, skipping, walking, and jogging. It will be simpler to maintain an exercise routine if you choose exercises you enjoy.

For parents

If you are the parent of an overweight or obese adolescent, you can assist them in making these small lifestyle adjustments. Throughout the process, assist them and provide constructive criticism. Motivate them by starting with modifications to your lifestyle, such as adopting a balanced diet and increasing your level of physical activity. Encourage them to change their diets for the better and keep them from turning into couch potatoes.

In conclusion, the advice provided above will help you shed 50 pounds quickly.

However, you shouldn't overwork your body when attempting to lose weight; starving yourself and doing strenuous exercises will harm your body more than they will help.

How would your life be if you were attractive and fit? You can get rid of all that extra weight in a matter of months if you act now.

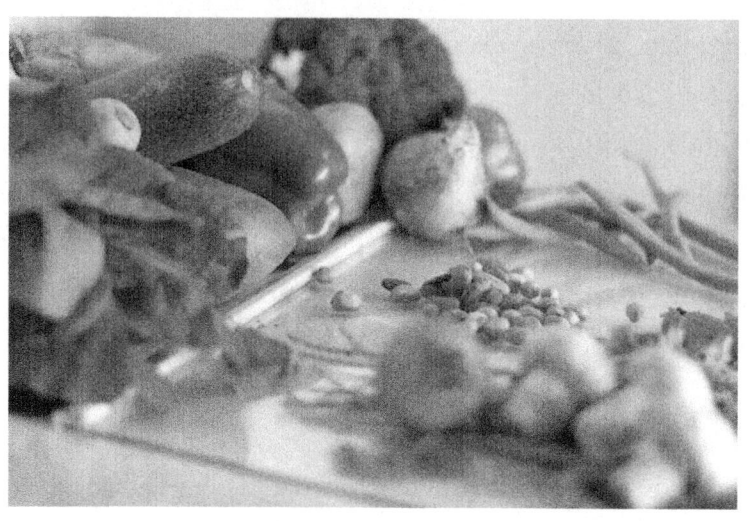

Teenage girls' extreme diets

Teenage girls' moods and looks can easily be lifted by diets and years are a time of rapid growth and high energy demands. Huge appetites result from this, which can be disastrous if the wrong foods are wolfed down.

Teenagers should make the time and effort to eat a healthy diet. A healthy body helps with annoying adolescent problems like acne and "puppy fat," but also makes girls happier and more attractive to boys. It's a universal truth that eating better will make you happier.

According to a recent study, teenage girls ate too much saturated fat, sugar, salt, and too few carbohydrates. Teenage girls are avoiding eating carbohydrates like rice, pasta, bread, and potatoes due to scary stories about them. This is absurd because teenagers need these foods for healthy development and growth. Well, a small serving of macaroni cheese with sliced tomato, salad greens, and cucumber would be the ideal healthy lunch option instead of a massive mountain of spaghetti dripping with high-fat meat sauce but the key is to consume "real food" sparingly.

A soda and fast-food burger for lunch will provide an adolescent with enough energy to last all day. However, a meal like this wouldn't have much in it that would help a teen's body grow. Only a few vitamins and minerals, if any at all, are present, but saturated fats abound. Fast food is acceptable if consumed in combination with healthy foods, but in the case of obesity, it should be the first casualty of the war on fat.

Vitamin deficiency is frequently a serious but unnoticed issue. Teenage girls' diets frequently don't contain enough iron. Red meat is the primary source of iron in food, but there are many other options as well, including dried fruit, bread, green leafy vegetables, and fortified cereals. Start the day with an apple, followed by a high-quality breakfast cereal (check the packet for added vitamins), chopped fruit, as well as a glass of orange juice on the side. Add a piece of whole-wheat toast to finish. Orange juice contains vitamin C, which is healthy in and of itself and aids in the body's absorption of other nutrients.

Teenage girls frequently lack calcium, which can cause issues later in life, particularly given the risk of osteoporosis. The nutrition consumed during the teenage years is crucial to this process because bones continue to grow and strengthen until the age of 30. Daily consumption of dairy products like milk and cheese is recommended. Teenage girls who are concerned about the fat content of dairy products can substitute low-fat milk and yogurt for it.

Teenage girls' diets must include these foods to function correctly:

- Pasta, rice, bread, breakfast cereals, potatoes, and couscous are starchy foods.
- Fruit and vegetables in abundance. Whatever you can manage.
- Two servings or more of protein Meat, fish, eggs, beans, pulses, and baked beans.
- 2-3 portions of dairy products like milk, cheese, and yogurt.
- Drinking 6 to 8 glasses of water each day is ideal (no soda, tea, or coffee).

Steer clear of all sodas, processed foods with added sugar, and fatty foods. Exercise a little while enjoying yourself by dancing, walking, running, or playing soccer. Teenage girls' diets will function best when combined with regular exercise.

Conclusion

People who are parents now or who will soon become parents undoubtedly worry and wonder how to raise their children. They'll also want more information on the kinds of things they should and shouldn't do when raising children of different ages. You will gain a lot from using child-rearing books, which are a great investment for anyone who wants to learn more about being a parent.

This book has provided some interesting information about parenting manuals for your daughter, but a lot of parenting manuals focus primarily on child development. The importance of proper development is emphasized because it will determine not only how well your children develop intellectually and socially but also how they will grow up. For instance, many scientific studies and parenting manuals claim that early exposure to music and art helps children develop better and increases their chances of becoming wiser, even while they are still in their mothers' wombs. Parenting books cover topics like how to teach your children about art and music, what types of music are best for learning and growth, and other elements that have a positive influence on a child's development.

Nutrition is another important topic in parenting books because it has an impact on children's physical and intellectual development. For their bodies to be properly nourished, to stay healthy, and to have a stronger resistance to viruses and illnesses, your children will need a lot of nutrients. The right types of food will support brain function, which has an impact on psychological development as well. Parenting manuals provide lists of foods that are suitable for kids of different ages and have the most minerals and vitamins for anxious parents. In addition, parenting books will discuss what foods to avoid or restrict.

Parenting books offer more than just advice for parents on how to raise their kids. They also emphasize how to deal with household problems that arise regularly. Many children exhibit negative behavior, especially when they are preschoolers and teenagers. Some traits don't call for immediate action; in the majority of cases, children would resolve their problems on their own and move past this stage. One particularly bad trait that is typical in children of all ages is stubbornness. Parenting manuals will provide you with tried-and-true methods to combat defiance and reduce this kind of behavior.

However, there are some extreme traits and tendencies that need to be addressed as soon as possible, and parents must use strategies that are appropriate for the age of their children. Children's books teach you how to avoid potentially dangerous situations like these and how to deal with them if they do occur. Yelling, threatening, carrying out the assault, and retaliation are not encouraged.

Naturally, child-rearing books discuss excellent behavior and how to praise and reward your girls and boys if they have been following your rules and carrying out their duties to the letter. One type of desirable behavior that all parents want their children to possess and exhibit responsibility. Child-rearing manuals frequently advise parents to develop responsibility skills, particularly when around their children. This would enable their boys and girls to understand and demonstrate it even as adults. Make sure your kids pick up after themselves, occasionally do the dishes, clean their rooms, and take care of their animals. These could be categorized as responsible behavior-promoting activities.

Self-esteem is a quality that everyone should possess, and it is important to start fostering it in children as soon as possible. When they start going to school and forming relationships with other girls and boys, having self-confidence and a sense of identity will be of great assistance to them. Furthermore, it has been found that girls and boys who are self-assured are happier, more outgoing, and frequently succeed in daily life. You could learn how to give your kids the self-esteem they need from parenting books.

Simply put, parenting manuals are created to assist you in learning about parenting, ways to prepare for it, and what to anticipate from the most demanding job you will ever have in your life. These parenting books cover a wide range of topics that you may or may not encounter, and they are very helpful for both new and seasoned fathers and mothers.

This book's contents are provided for informational purposes only and are not meant to be taken as medical advice. You should routinely seek medical advice and care from your doctor or another healthcare professional. Consult your doctor right away if you have any issues that worry your daughter.

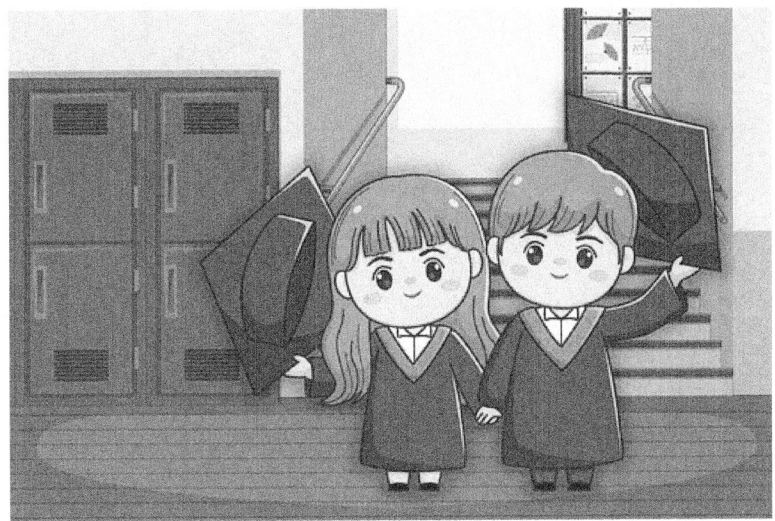

Thank you for getting and reading this book and I hope you get value. Cheers to your beautiful girl!

Printed in Great Britain
by Amazon